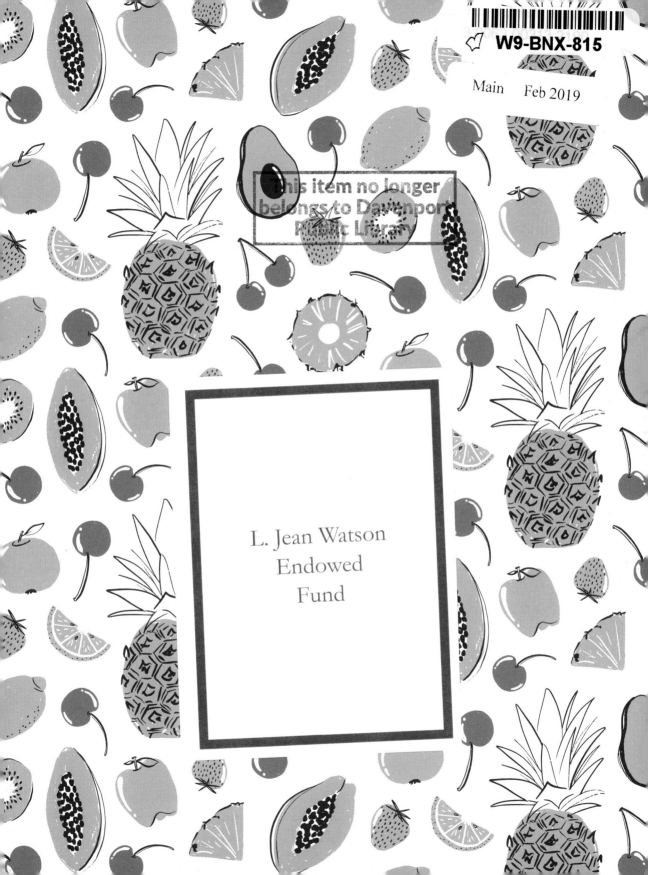

L. Jean Watson
Endowed
Fund

do what feels

good

HANNAH BRONFMAN

WITH SANDRA BARK

do what feels good

RECIPES, REMEDIES,
AND ROUTINES TO
TREAT YOUR BODY RIGHT

HARPER WAVE
An Imprint of HarperCollins*Publishers*

I want to dedicate

this book and the findings

of this process to my

GRANNY ANN

whose struggle, perseverance,

and resilience

inspire me every day.

you wanna

FLY

you got to give up the shit
that weighs you down.

—TONI MORRISON, *SONG OF SOLOMON*

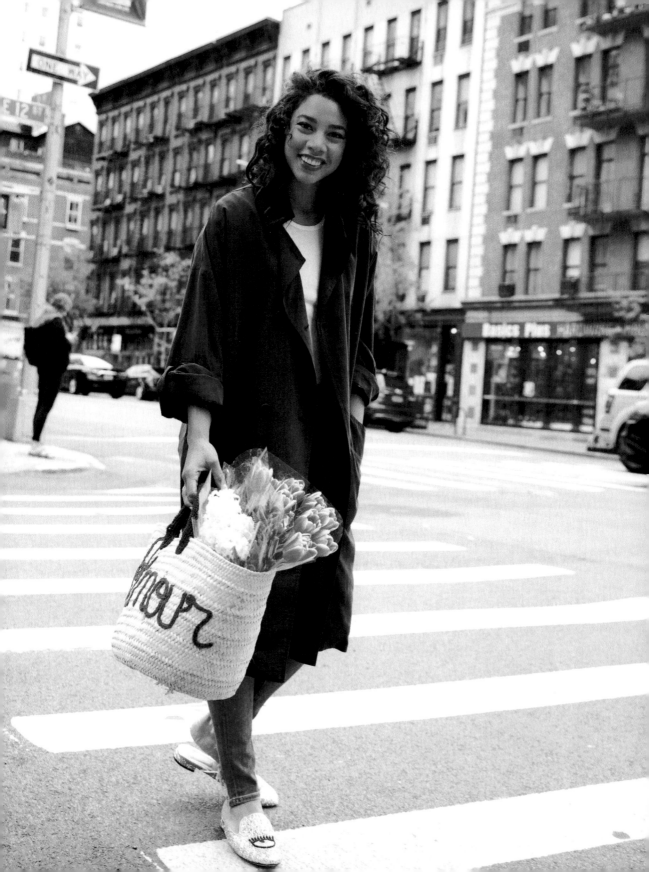

CONTENTS

do what feels
good

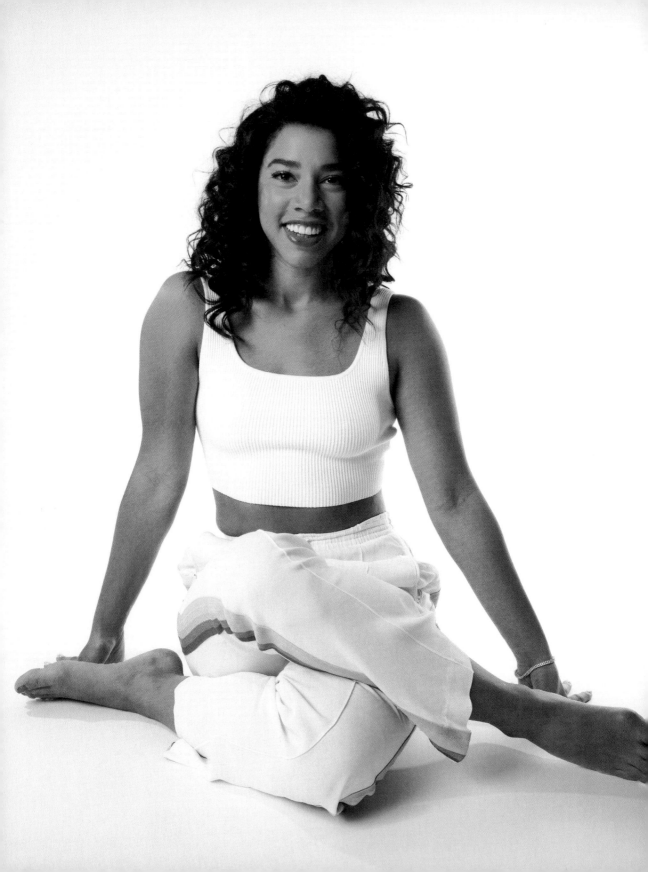

introduction

Hi, I'm Hannah. My friends call me HBFIT, which comes from the days when I started documenting my health journey on Instagram. I was a DJ who was just getting to know this world of wellness, and I would tag photos of all the smoothies and workouts and beauty products I was loving #hbfit. Over time, as health became more and more central in my life, the nickname stuck.

I love discovering everything new that is out there. Whatever's going on in fitness, food, and beauty, I want to try it and taste it. If it works for me, I'll usually write about it for HBFIT, the online community I launched so that women could share knowledge with each other in a welcoming, inclusive, zero-judgment, no-haters, pressure-free zone. I'm all about self-care and health from the perspective of what makes women feel good. I started the company because I wanted to talk about what I loved with other women who were feeling the same pressures and concerns that I was.

When I was growing up in New York City as a young, black, Jewish woman and going to ballet school, I spent a lot of time trying to understand why I didn't look like everyone else around me or why I was expected to. Maybe that's why I wanted to be an artist, so I could break out of the mold in some way.

In college, I studied sculpture in a small town where there was one local bar, and of course we hung out there as often as you would if you were twenty years old and there was only one place to go. One night I was chilling with my friend Henry, talking about how we were bored with the music they played at our one haunt. We were convinced we would be able to throw an epic party if they would only give us an aux cord and let all our friends into the bar.

So we told the owner. We said we would bring our own equipment and bring people with us, and he finally agreed to let us DJ a party. It wound up turning into a rager, and the owner asked us to throw a party every Thursday night going forward.

> If I was going to focus so much energy on my physical body, it couldn't be about meeting some societal idea of perfection.

That summer, at home in New York City, I made the rounds of the nightclubs to convince the managers or owners, whoever would talk to me, to let me play. I showed up and asked for a job every week until finally someone gave me a chance. Eventually other club owners heard about me, and I started getting some gigs.

I moved back to New York City in 2010. Jobs were scarce, and I couldn't afford a studio space and materials for sculpting, so I kept on DJing. I became a staple in the New York scene, and certainly one of the only black female DJs around. It was super fun and I met wildly cool people, but after three years I was tired and burned out. I couldn't continue living such a demanding nightlife—it was draining, mentally and physically. I'd started to lose touch with myself and the things that made me happy. I was no longer a morning person like I had been, I never worked out, and I usually didn't eat more than one meal a day. Honestly, I was a mess.

I was tired of feeling exhausted, so I began talking with experts about what

I could do to feel good. That was such a turning point for me. That was when I began trying all the good stuff—the newest trends and philosophies as well as the most ancient of human health secrets. That's when I buckled up and surrendered to my health journey.

WELLNESS ON MAIN

From that moment forward, I was all about transformation—my own kind of transformation. As a younger person I had struggled with body image and with my weight, and none of that struggle made me feel very good. If I was going to focus so much energy on my physical body, it couldn't be about meeting some societal idea of perfection. The motivation for my health journey needed to come from me and me alone, and my guiding philosophy—my goal—was to do things that would make me feel good. If restricting my eating made me feel anxious, I needed to listen to my body and eat more of what was good for me, less of what wasn't. (And also make sure to enjoy a burger once in a while.) If drinking milk made my stomach hurt, I needed to find ways of getting the richness and satisfaction of dairy without getting the cows and goats involved. If certain workouts felt like they were hurting my body, I would find the ones that strengthened it in a way that felt right for me.

I wanted to get to know myself, my body, and what I really liked and needed. I was willing to try anything to figure it out. I loved the trial and error of being a guinea pig, testing out the latest fads and learning from each experience what actually worked for me. As I progressed further and further into this growing space of wellness, I wanted to share all the cool stuff I was getting to try, so I started posting tips on Instagram. Insert hashtag hbfit.

What I found was that so many people had curiosity about the exact same things I did. My friends suddenly wanted to talk to me about health and wellness all the time. Everyone wanted to ask me about the crazy class I has just taken, or the colonic I'd just had, or the meal they saw me post on Instagram. They wanted to tell me what they were doing and trying and ask me for recommendations. Ultimately, though, what they were really asking me was what they were supposed to do and how they were supposed to feel. This gave me a new sense of purpose. Suddenly people were looking to me for answers. I wanted to arm myself

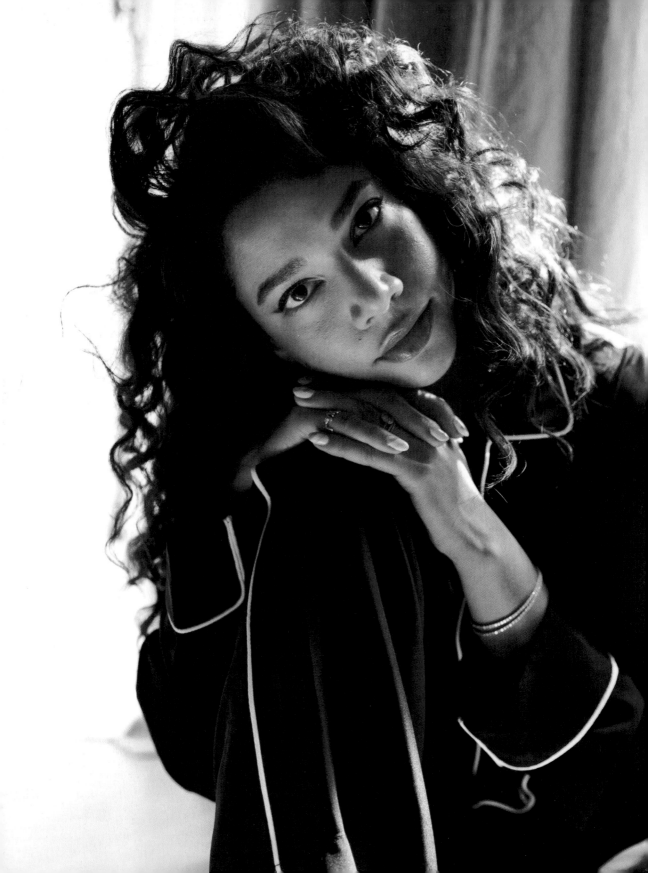

with the best information I could find and share it far and wide.

When I started HBFIT, I wanted to make a space to talk about the rituals that give us energy and that make us feel confident. I wanted to create a resource for the supplements and creams and foods and movements that help to heal what ails us—to balance our hormones and our moods, to clear our skin and our minds. I wanted to talk about the stuff that worked for me, but I also wanted to talk about why we are all so obsessed with "wellness" in the first place. Is it because we want what's best for ourselves, or because we're aspiring to achieve someone else's vision of who we should be? There's a lot of pressure to do the "cool" thing or the "right" thing, but what if those things aren't right for you? It's great to have so many options to try out, but at the end of the day it's also overwhelming. Becoming healthy shouldn't hurt and shouldn't stress you out. The journey shouldn't suck. It should be fun and different and make you feel all sorts of good, strong, and empowered.

That doesn't mean that sometimes a hard workout doesn't kick my ass. It usually does, and that's a sign to me that I'm getting stronger. And it doesn't mean that I'll put into practice what I've learned every single day. There will be days when I just want pancakes for lunch (this literally happened while we were shooting the recipes for this book). There will be weeks I'm traveling so much that I don't get the sleep or hydration that I know is optimal for me to feel my best. Here's the thing: All of this stuff is okay. Nights I stay out too late. It happens. Sometimes it even feels good (I mean, the cocktails—pages 206–219—are pretty ridiculous). But more often than not, when I'm off my routine, it feels the opposite of good. And so I'm guided to choices that return me to a state of feeling good.

Today, I only want the best around me because I am a busy woman and there is so much to do. I'm still a DJ and travel around the world spinning tunes for fashion brands, publishers, tech companies, and much more. I'm always investigating what is new and worthy when it comes to wellness trends so I can create content for HBFIT, for Instagram, and for YouTube, for brands I love.

I guess you could say I'm a Renaissance woman seeking opportunity at every corner. Because of what I do, I am able to gain access to so many incredible experts and thought leaders in the wellness space. And I want to share what I've learned!

I wrote this book for the same reason I started sharing my journey and discoveries online: because it's my mission to live my life as the happiest and healthiest version of myself, and to share what I've learned with the people that I care about. The way we nurture ourselves matters, and the way we support each other matters, too. I'll do anything I can to promote a healthy body image or to give a young woman more reasons to love herself.

For centuries women have been subjected to so many expectations about how we should look and act and speak, and I say screw that. The only person who gets to set expectations for me is ME. The only person who gets to set the bar for you is YOU. We want to break societal norms as twenty-first-century women, and that starts with knowing who we are, what we deserve, and how to take care of ourselves and one another with love, compassion, and honor. If you want to be a superhero, you need to identify your superpower. You need to give your attention to the things that make you feel incandescent.

Good health is a gift, but it should not be a privilege. Everyone deserves to feel good.

Everything I know about beauty, health, fitness, and food, I learned by trying. Like so many of us, I grew up surrounded by unhealthy body images and body issues both at home and out in the world, and I had to work hard to change the way I see myself and define what's beautiful. My approach to beauty and health is based on self-acceptance and self-expression, because I think a woman is most beautiful and radiates well-being when she embraces her individuality. You are not the same as anyone else, and that is part of your superpower.

Do What Feels Good is a resource for self-care. It is not a diet book, it is not a how-to guide, it is not an instruction manual for how to be like me. It is a compendium of the best advice and supportive information I know of. It's the information I rely on daily, and information I hope is helpful to you on your own health journey. In every one of our lives, there will be days that we struggle and days that we feel amazing. I'm not here tell you what you "should" be doing every day;

I just want to offer you the basics to do whatever you want in the healthiest way that you can.

Here's what you'll find in this book: an approach to self-care that is holistic, hedonistic, and real. Just to give you a little preview, we'll learn from the experts about the mind-body connection and how paying attention to physical symptoms can help us understand what our bodies need to feel good (spoiler alert: it's different for every one of us!); we'll look at the hot new trend of adaptogenic herbs (although these herbs have been used for centuries) and how they can help the body adapt to stress and achieve hormonal balance; we'll learn why a healthy gut makes for a healthy body (and clear skin); we'll try out some of my favorite feel-good tonics and homemade masks; and I'll share my go-to recipes for everything from breakfast to snacks to cake to cocktails, because eating delicious food is a super-important part of feeling food.

According to the World Health Organization, being "healthy" isn't just about being disease-free. It's about feeling good physically, mentally, and socially. Your health is the most powerful tool at your disposal. It is at the foundation of everything you are doing and will do. Good health is a gift, but it should not be a privilege. Everyone deserves to feel good. That's something I want for myself, and for you.

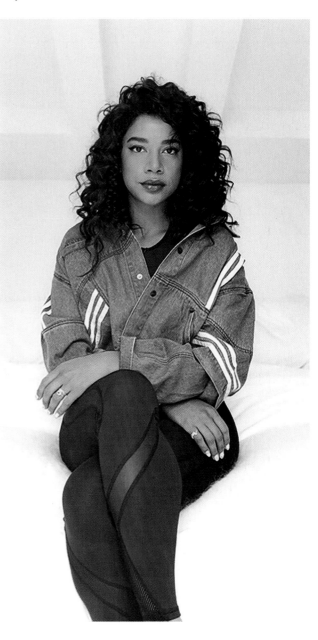

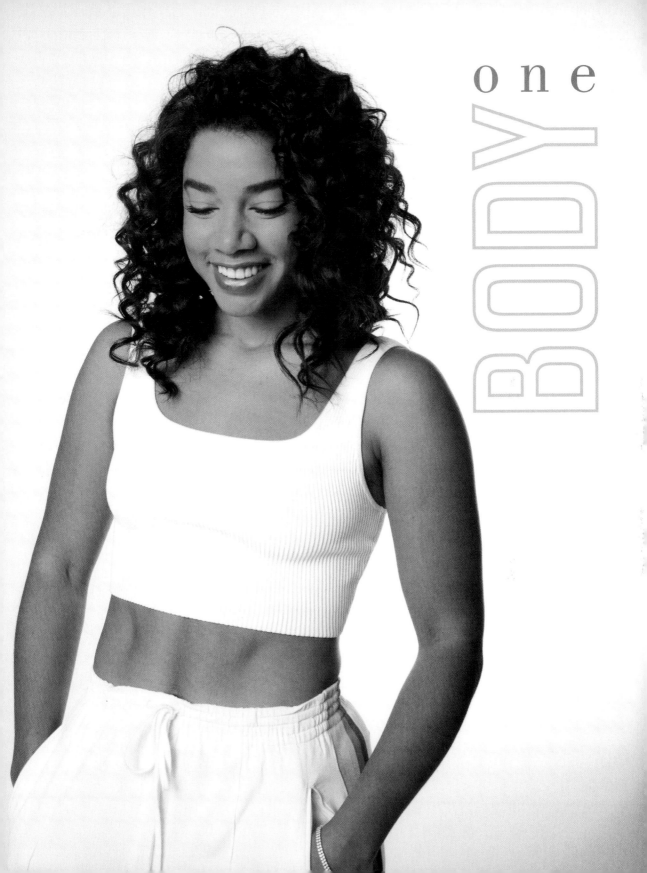

one

BODY

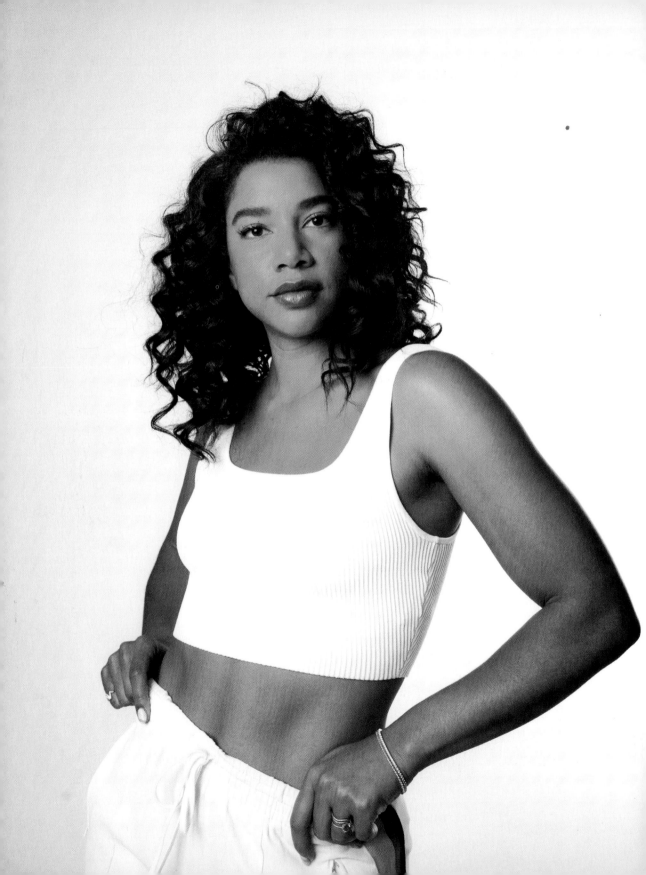

everybody HAS AN OPINION

TUNING OUT THE HATERS

The first time I got my period, I was away at performing arts camp for the summer. I went to study ballet for seven weeks amid the pine trees and crisp summer air instead of the heated fumes of New York City. Since it was an all-girls camp, you might imagine that someone could have taken me aside and offered an encouraging talk and a positive perspective on the changes my body was about to experience. But no. The announcement that I was bleeding was not met with a warm and friendly arm around my shoulder and a loving speech about the beauty in becoming a woman. This wasn't that kind of place.

It was not a place where we ate s'mores and told ghost stories around a roaring fire. It was not a place where you were told that you were beautiful just as you are or that you had your own gifts to discover and appreciate. It was a place where we danced for nine hours a day internalizing messed-up ideas about "health" and female beauty.

If beauty was based on a typical ballerina's body type, everything about my body—about me—felt wrong. That's because everything I thought about myself was based on what I imagined other people were thinking about me.

What I remember from the day I stepped out of the bathroom stall with the excitement that I was finally a woman was this: someone shoving a tampon at me and saying something along the lines of *Stick that up there and make it snappy, because we're going to be late for class. And don't even think about going to the infirmary to deal with cramps, because the nurse isn't having it.*

Everything I thought about myself was based on what I imagined other people were thinking about me.

It was made very clear to all of us at this camp that skinny was good and fat was bad. And now I had my period. This was embarrassing because somewhere along the line I had internalized the message that heavier girls got their periods earlier. So getting my period at twelve years old, before most of the other girls at camp, made me worry that I was fat. I was just a kid going through a totally natural change, and I wasn't encouraged to process what it meant in the larger sense of going through puberty, or to take even a minute to call my mom. How was I supposed to come to terms with my maturing body—which I was kind of excited about—when the signals I was getting from the people around me were that I should be worried or disappointed?

It's crazy to me now to think that I was developing from a girl to a woman in the context of an ideology that suggested that NOT getting your period was a good thing. But that's what happened. And so I felt even more self-conscious about my first period than I might have otherwise. Because instead of being told that it was completely normal, instead of feeling like I was part of something bigger, the flow of life itself, instead of getting to be excited that my body was changing, I took it as just another sign that there was something wrong with me, that I wasn't good enough, and that I had to do something to "fix" myself.

The world of ballet as I experienced it was all about image. I was surrounded by girls who thought it was normal to starve themselves to try to fit into this standard of what a dancer should look like, while still having enough energy to perform grueling pirouettes on repeat. There was a physical ideal, and it was made very clear to us. It would be best, we all knew, if we were willowy, long-legged, and gazelle-like. I didn't think I looked anything like that, and I kept feeling as though I was falling short.

And so that summer I was trying to lose weight. In fact, I was eating significantly less than what I would have normally been eating as an adolescent person. I can't say that it was my idea or that I was the only one. There was plenty of pressure to eat as little as possible so you could weigh as little as possible. Staying away from bread and carbs in general was the first thing I learned about "dieting." Early in the summer, at dinner, I was hungry and wanted to have a second course, but the looks I got from my peers said *Don't do it*.

When I think about it now, I see that because I didn't know better, and because of the lack of open communication and education, I absorbed unhealthy habits, language, and thoughts that eventually my whole body was listening to.

KEEP THE FAMILY CLOSE

The pressure to be thin didn't only exist at camp—it was part of my daily life. I grew up in a loving family that loved food. Food was ever present in our house. Someone was always cooking, there was always something good on the stove or on the counter or wrapped in aluminum foil in the fridge, just waiting for you. Also ever present was the obsession with being slim, and so any extra portions came with extra side-eye. And not just looks. Comments.

If there was a cake around and you even thought about reaching for more than one slice, there it was, floating through the air like a verbal slap.

"You're going to get fat."

Ouch.

What a confusing way to be in the

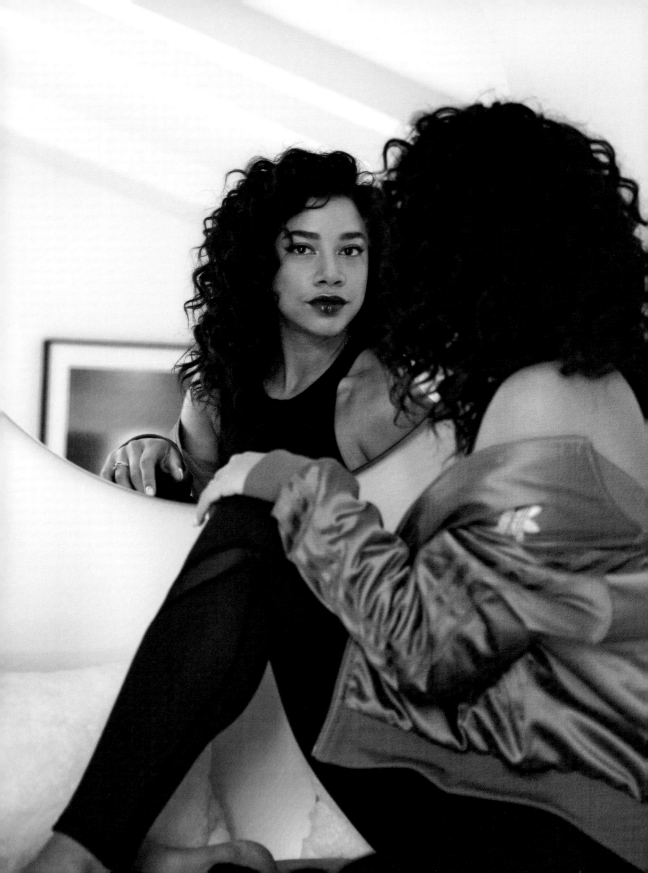

world. Where you have enough, but you can't enjoy it, because it comes with a warning: This enjoyment will ruin you, will ruin your life, will make you disgusting to other people and to yourself. My house was a place where doing something I loved—eating delicious food—felt dangerous and shameful. Enjoyment was like a form of self-torture. It's a terrible thing when our human need to eat and enjoy our food gets mixed up with judgments about our bodies. Because hating your body comes too easily and pretty close to hating yourself.

And so I was always worried that I was too fat. I worried that I was eating too much, so I would eat less. Or I would eat a normal amount, feel terrible about it, and then undereat to compensate or soothe. Instead of thinking of myself as young and growing, or strong and getting stronger, instead of seeing myself as worthy of love and respect, I thought I was weak and I

felt ashamed because I wasn't as thin as I should be.

It took me a long time to get to a place where I could really love and enjoy my food, where I could understand that it was there to nourish me and help me achieve my goals, not somehow keep me from them. Now I know that hunger is nothing to be afraid of—it is my body's way of communicating what it needs to feel good. I know that food is good for me, that food nourishes me, that I can use it to nurture and care for myself. I know that I am allowed to *enjoy* eating, that food can and should be pleasurable. Just because I am a woman doesn't mean that I need to pretend like I'm never hungry or that my hunger is something to apologize for.

But as a young person, I had a hard time listening to the quiet wisdom of my body. That voice was drowned out by a lot of louder ones that told me food was the enemy.

THROUGH GENERATIONS

My paternal grandmother and I were very close. When it comes to body image, I guess you could say that she was my teacher. But not in the way you might think.

My grandmother was always a beautiful woman. She was a German Jew who

was very fair-skinned; I was conscious that we didn't look alike, and as a little girl, I was a bit scared of her. I always thought of her as glamorous and poised, but she had an air of snootiness that made me feel like I wasn't refined enough for her. I mean, at eight years old, who the hell is refined?

My parents got divorced when I was two. I always knew that none of my grandparents had approved of my parents' marriage, but once my parents had children, my paternal grandmother came around and was involved in our lives. To a degree! We all knew she didn't really like kids. When it was just my sister and brother, before I was born, my grandmother came over for dinner one night. My dad was running a music label at the time, and when they called about a new act he needed to go see, he asked if she would stick around and watch the kids. She agreed, but she made him promise not to tell his siblings. She had no intentions of being an on-call babysitter.

Granny Ann was a complicated woman, but stories about her were legend in my family. Growing up, I always heard about her badass achievements. She sailed around the world with her best friend and lost two fingers in a boating accident. Her best friend, a woman, was also her lover. That is not a part of the story I knew about as a girl, but it made me feel even more in awe of her when I was older.

We also knew about some of her cutting one-liners. Like the time she was out to dinner with friends and a waiter of-fered her the bread basket. Her response? "Never serve bread to a Loeb" (that was her last name). It was kind of funny, was a lot unkind, and betrayed volumes about how uncomfortable she felt in her own skin.

While I was a bit in awe of her, I could also sense something fragile in her, and I always felt like I was walking on eggshells around her. As I got older and learned more about her, I discovered that she'd had a twin brother who was born with cerebral palsy. Her parents told her it was her fault, something she she'd done to him in the womb. Because her brother had to be on medication from a young age, they put her on medication as well. But she didn't need those meds, and they actually damaged her body.

When she and my grandpa divorced, she had five children who ranged in age from eleven to nineteen. Alone and unable to cope with the demands of mothering five kids, she would lock herself in her room for days just drinking and crying. She didn't have anyone there to support her. And she didn't know how to support herself.

My grandma was always petite, but by the time I was a teenager, she had become tiny, fragile, and very sick. It wasn't until I was older that I learned my grandmother was depriving herself of the nutrients she needed because she suffered from anorexia. It was challenging to witness her behavior because it was so second nature to her. It blew my mind to think that she'd struggled her entire life with her emotional relationship to food and to herself.

Watching my grandma suffer was painful on many levels, and it hit home for me in a profound way. I saw firsthand what can happen when other people's standards of beauty become your own. At the same time that I was struggling with food and trying to attain some imaginary status of perfection (I think we're all familiar with what the world expects from young women), I was also seeing the tragic outcome of such views. I was seeing how you could internalize dangerous and damaging messages and carry them with you for a lifetime. I was seeing how much pain my grandmother endured, mentally and physically. I wanted something different for myself, and I knew my grandmother also wanted that for me. That's the gut feeling that I had watching her deteriorate before my eyes.

> I saw firsthand what can happen when other people's standards of beauty become your own.

I was with my grandmother when she passed away. At twenty, I felt very clearly that though she wasn't able to achieve it for herself, one thing my grandmother was really good at was telling me to be happy. I had felt as a young child that I wasn't refined enough for her, but that wasn't it at all. Through conversations we had when she was ill, I realized that she wanted me to be comfortable being myself. She didn't want me to struggle with societal standards of beauty the way she did. She wanted me to embrace my body, my race, and my power as a woman.

Ultimately, she inspired me to be vocal about the issues she was never able to resolve for herself. Anorexia is an extreme example of what can happen when we make choices about our health that are not based on how we feel but rather what society says we should look like. My grandmother's story is one about how sick we can become when we neglect our inner voice and don't treat ourselves with love and respect.

Granny Ann is one reason why I have made it my mission to take care of

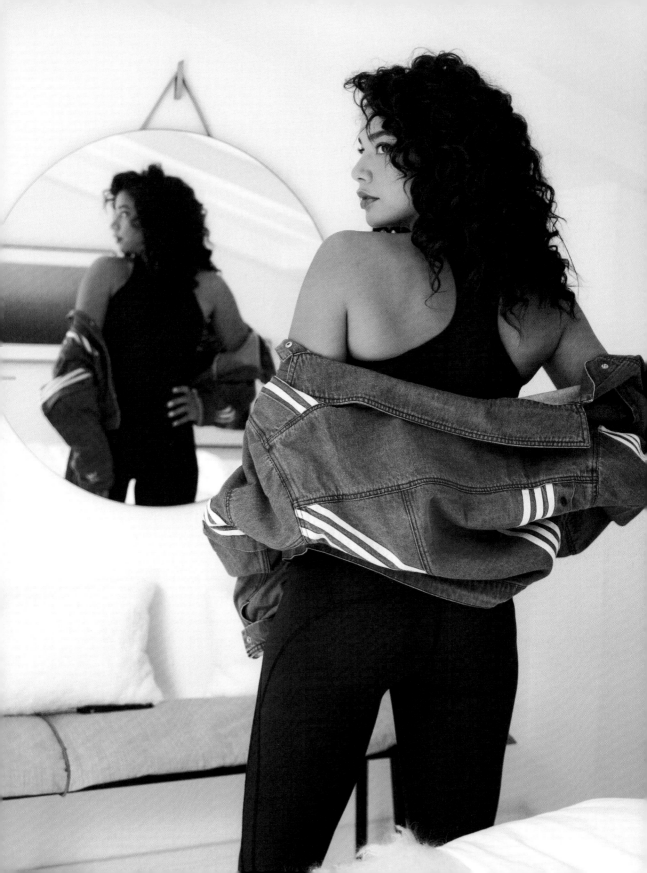

my own health. The other reason is my mother, who has worked so hard to give me a healthy view of myself. When my grandmother was sick, my mom and I talked a lot about how upset it made me that Granny felt so trapped and so angry in her body. My mom always encouraged me to listen to my feelings and be vocal about my beliefs. My mother is a woman who is extremely in tune with her spirit, who studied meditation since she was in her twenties and taught me about chakras when I was just a little girl. She has long been a source of positive body behavior and always did what made her feel good. Her messages still echo in my ears.

That's the kind of support I want to have on replay. It's why I want to spread the message far and wide about what it means to love and accept your body, to listen to and respect and nourish your body, and to let feeling good lead you.

F*CK THE THIGH GAP

If you could change anything about yourself, what would it be?

As I considered how our ideals of beauty and body image are formed, how we are all affected by other people's standards and beliefs, I began initiating open and honest conversations with the women in my life (beautiful, smart, talented women, I might add) and asking them this one simple question.

The first place most of us went to was the physical—to what we imagine other people see when they look at us. Nobody wished for a stronger singing voice, the ability to run a marathon, a higher salary—at first. In order to get there, to what we *really* wanted, to what we were passionate about, we had to muddle through all of our insecurities about our physical forms.

It starts out small. It's so easy to say, I wish I was thinner, I wish I was taller, I hate my double chin, I hate my arms, I hate my curly hair/straight hair. All those minor imperfections, those wrinkles, that saggy stomach, the hair that's too big, the hair that's too flat. Too tall, too short. Ugly feet. Stubby nails. It's crazy-making, and it is crazy to me that we give away so much of our power as women in an attempt to conform to some ideal of physical perfection that is subjective and largely unobtainable. This is something we have to unlearn so that we can get to the good stuff. So we can take that question deeper. What would you REALLY change?

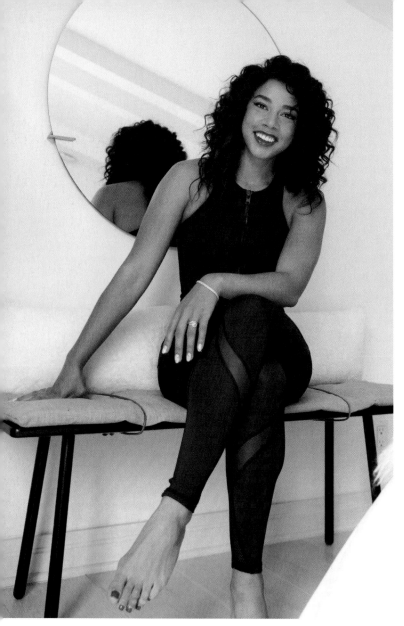

dards swirling around us affect the way we see ourselves—and why we should give those misplaced, outdated attitudes the finger. Because that's not the only gap that impacts how we feel in our lives and about ourselves every day. There are gaps in education and equality. There is a wage gap, where women earn less than men, where white women earn more than black women. The thigh gap should be the least of our concerns. And yet these social and political issues are not entirely separate from the body issues.

Beauty is political. The thigh gap and the wage gap are related. Why do we put certain pressures on ourselves? Why so much encouragement from the media to worry about my body instead of my salary?

It seems like more and more, the person you want to be like just wants to be like someone else who wants to be like someone else. Does anybody want to be themselves? "What do we want and why?" is the question we all have to ask. Whom do you give power to when it comes to questions about your body? Are you choosing the right heroes?

But the thing is, unlearning is not so easy, and it isn't just personal. It's cultural. It's political. It's bigger than we are, and we need to see it to rise above it.

One of the most-viewed articles on HBFIT was called "F*ck the Thigh Gap." It was about how all these "beauty" stan-

do what feels good

It's very hard to see the stuff of our times. But take a moment to think about the history of beauty and just wind back the clock from where we are now for a second. The idea of beauty changes with every generation—but it always falls within societal norms. These ideas conform to who is at the top at that moment, what that person and their children look like. It's very subtle while it's happening, because everybody who feels bad just keeps quiet and buys in, and colors their hair, or straightens their hair, or pads their bra, or gets plastic surgery. And the subliminal messaging becomes what you see around you all of the time.

If you look at ads from the '50s, you can see the standard so clearly—it's all housewives with small waists and A-line skirts and men bossing them around in a way that screams "misogyny" today. Go back further to where women had to wear corsets. For so long, women have been asked to make themselves smaller.

In this era, in this country, we are conditioned to think that a thin appearance is more beautiful than a curvy body. We are constantly fed images that show us that being thin will take us further in society. How many hours have you spent looking in the mirror trying to suck in and imagine what you would look like with a different body? Those are the kinds of pressures that my grandma absorbed. Those are the pressures that led to so much of her suffering.

Then there's the pressure of looking different. Because historically white people had the privilege and power, because we have spent centuries watching women with lighter skin get ahead, women whose skin is darker, who were not born looking like Barbie, have continuously tried to emulate those types of images. This is psychologically stressful, all of the time. How can you feel good on the inside when the world is always telling you that there is something damaged about your outside?

I'll tell you this: It isn't you who needs to change. It's the ideas around you that

> Beauty is political. The thigh gap and the wage gap are related. Why so much encouragement from the media to worry about my body instead of my salary?

need reshaping so that they can fit you, instead of the other way around.

I reject the idea that we are all supposed to look the same and that we are supposed to be uncomfortable or unhealthy in order to fit into someone else's idea of what is beautiful. I think we are supposed to look exactly like ourselves, and that we can adorn our bodies with whatever clothes, makeup, or style we like if it makes us feel good. It's your right to stand out, to take up space.

When we get swept up by emotional waves about our perceived physicality based on other people's perceptions, that's when we start to drown. We devote so much energy to what we look like on the outside that we barely have the energy or space to look inward, which is where we need to focus in order to thrive and achieve our *actual* goals, not just our #bodygoals.

And so everything that comes next in this book comes with this caveat: Your definition of and journey to health is yours alone. In these pages I want to share with you what I have learned through the experience of living in my body, but in no way do I want to add to the pressure we already feel to be better/prettier/thinner/sexier/fitter/healthier. Consider this book an à la carte menu, a choose-your-own-adventure resource to getting to know your body a little better.

What I don't want for you is pressure. What I do want for you to have is energy throughout the day. Enthusiasm to share with your family and friends. Dedication to your work and interests and all the things you love to do. Confidence in yourself. That all starts with a routine and a lifestyle that you create for yourself with consciousness, kindness, and love.

Everything stems from how you feel. And I want you to feel incredible.

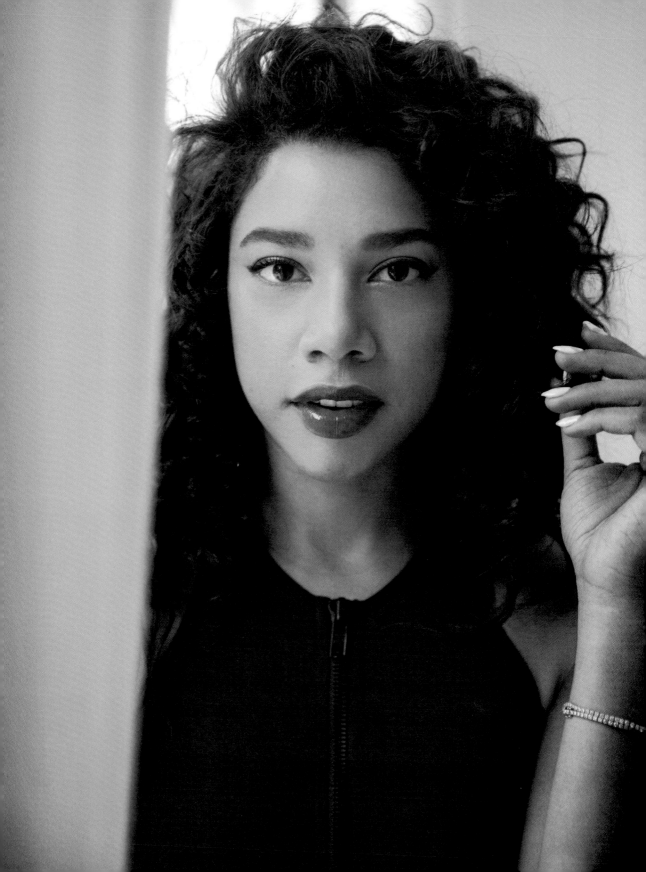

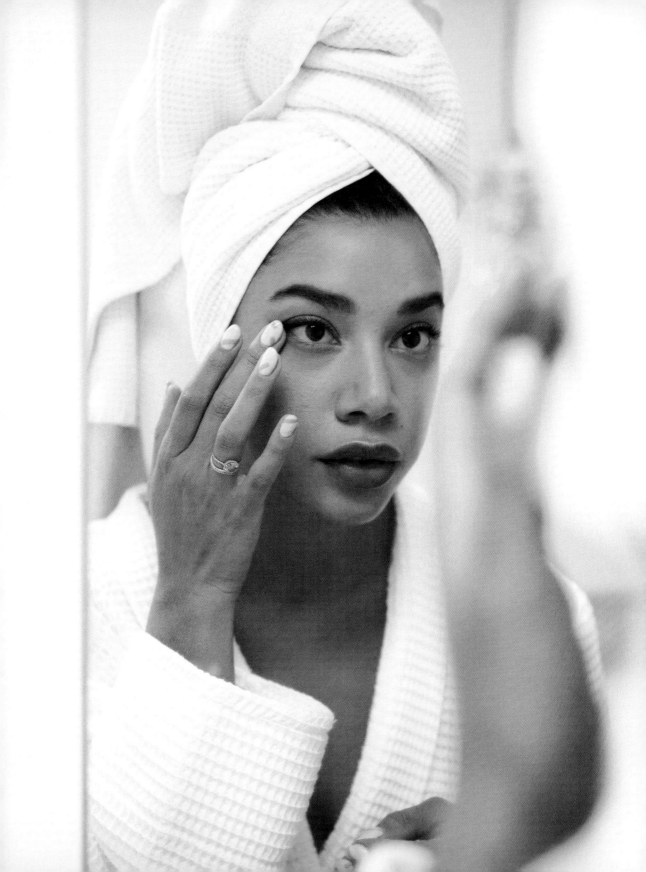

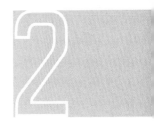

listen to YOUR BODY

YOUR SKIN TELLS A STORY

When I was in my early twenties and DJing clubs, nighttime was when everything happened. I would be up all night working, and then around 5 a.m. my friends and I would hit up a diner or some other random restaurant that was open really late and eat a massive breakfast to soak up the booze. I'd go home and pass out, sleeping all day, only to get up and eat whatever was around on the way out the door to get to the club to spin, and the cycle continued. There were cocktails and there was dancing and there were late-night dinners and early breakfasts and then back to sleep till the next round. When I look at pictures from those days, it looks like I'm having fun, which I was.

But what you don't see are the hungover mornings and days of just feeling like shit. You also don't see that underneath the makeup, my skin was a mess, because I was having a series of terrible breakouts.

I wasn't into feeling like shit, but I figured that just came with the territory. I wasn't into the breakouts. So I went to the dermatologist's office, and the doctor put me on a course of antibiotics. But my skin didn't clear. I kept putting on makeup and going back to the dermatologist, who would give me another course of antibiotics, and then another. And each time, my skin didn't clear. But my stomach started hurting, and I got my first yeast infection.

Now that I understand more about the connection between my insides and my outsides, none of this seems surprising. Physical issues have a tendency to compound if we don't get to the root cause. I wasn't eating well, I was ignoring all my symptoms except for the ones that were showing up on my face, and I was giving responsibility for my health to someone else, who thought the solution was medication. Something had to give. I needed—I deserved!—a better way.

Physical issues have a tendency to compound if we don't get to the root cause.

And I found one when a friend referred me to Dr. Gabrielle Francis, a holistic physician and the author of *The Rock Star Remedy*. Dr. Francis has toured with some of the biggest names in music. Her job is to keep her clients healthy and feeling well while they're on the road, in a new city every night performing high-energy sets, and partying like . . . well, rock stars. If anyone could understand my lifestyle, she could.

Dr. Francis gave me a whole bunch of tests to establish what was happening and what could help me. She did a saliva test. She did a food allergy test. She asked me a lot of questions about my gut and how often I was going to the bathroom and what I was eating and how all of it made me feel.

Dr. Francis turned out to be a body whisperer. She listened so closely that she found the root cause of a lot of my problems: I had something called leaky gut syndrome. This is a condition where the "gut"—your digestive tract—develops microscopic tears from a combination of food choices and lifestyle factors. Foods like grains, added sugars, and conventional dairy, for example, irritate the gut. Caffeine, alcohol, stress, and antibiotics further degrade the gut lining and wipe out the healthy microbes that live in the gut (more on that soon).

When holes form in your gut wall, the unfortunate side effect is that particles from inside the gut leak into your bloodstream, where they are then carried throughout your body. This provokes an immune response, because those particles are actually toxins meant to be eliminated in your stool—they don't belong in your blood! The immune system senses a menace and launches a response to protect you—but in this case, all it really does is create widespread inflammation and make things worse. That's why leaky gut is often linked with autoimmune diseases. Symptoms of leaky gut range from digestive issues to brain fog to skin problems.

Dr. Francis said that I needed to start repairing my digestive system so that my body could digest food, extract the nutrients it needed, and get rid of what it didn't need.

Finally, I had an approach that didn't come in the form of a pill. This one was based on listening to my body! The program Dr. Francis suggested for me included nutrient-rich shakes and lists of foods that could help heal my gut and those that would trigger inflammation. It was a complete change as far as how I was going to eat, and it required a fair amount of planning. It wasn't like I was going to do a ten-day course and—boom!—my gut problems would be solved. This was going to take time, discipline, accountability, and a proactive approach. I was going to have to start listening to what all of my organs were trying to tell me—including my skin.

BALANCED BODY, BALANCED SKIN

Dr. Francis suggested that I talk with Monica Watters, a holistic healer and skincare expert.

When I first met Monica, I could tell how passionate she was about her craft. The woman has skin like porcelain, and she radiates confidence. Monica uses several diagnostic tools including face map-

ping, a technique based on Traditional Chinese Medicine (TCM) and Ayurvedic medicine. Part of the philosophy of both of these medical systems is that the health of your skin, your only external organ, is a direct reflection of the health of your internal organs.

Traditional Chinese Medicine originated thousands of years ago, when the people of the Chinese royal court received treatments to improve and preserve their health and beauty. The teachings of TCM suggest that true beauty comes from the inside out because your skin mirrors your body condition.

The ancient medical system of Ayurveda is also thousands of years old and was developed in India as a study of the science of life around the idea of energy flow. In Ayurvedic tradition, life energy, or Prana, is thought to be constantly moving through our bodies. When our chakras, or energy centers, are blocked, we become imbalanced, and illness results. Ayurvedic medicine teaches us that nourishing foods and herbs can heal and restore balance, and that every individual's physiology is unique.

Breakouts, dull or flushed skin, red or swollen eyes—all of these symptoms are clues that can be interpreted to understand what your body is trying to tell you about its current state. When Monica sees those irritations, she is also seeing the underlying hormone imbalance or nutrition deficiency that is the root of the issue. She often asks questions about your cycle, your bowel movements, and your water intake, as all of these things are related to the health and appearance of your skin.

At the time I saw Monica, I was having visibly bad breakouts, inflammation, and congestion. Within minutes of examining and touching my skin, Monica went into full detail about what she thought was going on. She was the skin detective I was looking for. My daily choices were literally written all over my face, and she had the tools to understand how I could heal.

HOW TO READ YOUR FACE

When Monica would stare at my face, looking for clues, I would stare back, wondering what she was seeing when she looked at me. I asked her to show me what she was doing and what she was thinking about as she inspected my forehead, and she shared a face map with me that looked a lot like the one I've made for you here!

Your face is an intricate structure, with bones, muscles, nerves, and arteries, all delicately and precisely arranged so that you look like you. Your face has 43 muscles, and it can use those to make up to 10,000 micro-expressions to let the world know how you feel. It also holds valuable clues as to what's going on inside of you.

small intestines, bladder,
and gall bladder

liver and spleen

kidneys,
adrenals, and
joints

lungs and
respiratory
system

heart, circulation,
and blood

reproductive system,
lymphatic system, and
hormones

We've all woken up with puffy eyes due to not enough sleep, too much alcohol or too much salt. In TCM and Ayurvedic teachings, the appearance of the skin, face, eyes, nose, and jaw can give trained practitioners insights into your health.

As you can see, from the face map and chart, each part of your face corresponds to your internal organs. It is the quality of your skin in those areas that offers clues about what is happening inside your body. Once you know more about your individual chemistry, you can develop a routine that is in line with your needs.

UPPER

FOREHEAD: small intestines, bladder, and gall bladder.

Issues may be due to dehydration, stress, or digestion.

BETWEEN THE EYEBROWS: liver and spleen.

Issues may be due to anxiety, anger/rage, undigested emotions, alcohol, dairy, sugar, or too much salt.

EYES: kidneys, adrenals, and joints.

Issues may be due to adrenal exhaustion, dehydration, food allergies, medications, caffeine, or lack of sleep.

MIDDLE

CHEEKS: lungs and respiratory system.

Issues may be due to allergies, poor absorption, candida overgrowth, difficulty metabolizing and assimilating foods, or dental issues such as gingivitis or bleeding gums.

NOSE: heart, circulation, and blood.

Issues may be due to poor circulation, high blood pressure, bacterial overgrowth, acid reflux, or inflammation.

LOWER

CHIN AND JAW: reproductive system, lymphatic system, and hormones.

Issues may be due to toxin buildup, sluggish lymphatics, stress, menstrual cycle, or perimenopause.

FEED YOUR SKIN

Monica's evaluation of my situation basically echoed what Dr. Francis had told me. We talked about how much sugar I was eating, because too much sugar, along with caffeine and alcohol, can lead to systemic inflammation. And so another aha moment clicked for me.

Inflammation is an important physical response that can keep you healthy, because inflammatory responses are what spring to action to help heal the damage when you get a bruise or a cut. This is called acute inflammation, because it subsides pretty quickly once the job is done. But sometimes inflammation is triggered not by bumps and bruises but by your diet. And in this case—if you're eating the same foods most of the time—the inflammation becomes chronic. Chronic inflammation can lay the groundwork for a number of serious health issues, including diseases like cancer. So it was really important for me to learn how to keep my blood sugar stable and prevent my body from being chronically inflamed.

Since processed foods have a ton of added sugar, I needed to get back to eating more fruits and vegetables and lean proteins. I started thinking more seriously about how food is fuel and how we should power our bodies with nutritious food. That was when I started to get really into cooking for myself at home and developing the cooking style that I still rely on today to keep myself and my husband, Brendan, in fighting shape.

Monica taught me that once I was properly feeding myself, I would give my skin a chance to recover and become supple and radiant. When I realized that what I was eating was affecting my glow, I was excited to change things up and feel (and see) a difference. I didn't need to give up everything I loved. I just needed to make more considered choices so that I could leave guilt and regret behind in favor of total food bliss. The cool thing is that being a hedonist and being a health nut can sometimes be one and the same, which is probably one of the best things I've learned along my health journey!

GLOW FOODS

Here are a few of my favorite beauty goods. These are the magic potions that helped heal my gut, restore my hormone balance, and give me back my glow!

- **green tea** is high in antioxidants and polyphenols (aka wrinkle-fighters). It's also got some caffeine, so if you're easing off of coffee, it's a great choice for a morning beverage with just enough kick.
- **raw dark chocolate,** the food of the gods, is packed full of antioxidants, catechins, and procyanidin. The properties in dark chocolate help to keep the skin looking fresh and youthful.
- **red wine** is full of anti-inflammatory flavonoids and resveratrol, a compound that helps neutralize the damaging effects of free radicals, and thus offers anti-aging and anti-cancer benefits.
- **berries** contain anthocyanins, which protect your skin's collagen, and vitamin C, which is needed for making collagen in the first place.[1]
- **green vegetables,** especially spinach for selenium, is good for your skin's elasticity, and dark green vegetables like kale, broccoli, brussels sprouts, collards and other leafy greens, and arugula, are all high in vitamin E, which protects skin from free radicals caused by sun damage.[2]
- **cucumbers and celery** are chock-full of vitamins, minerals, antioxidants, and vitamins A and K. Antioxidants protect the skin from UV damage, and vitamin A helps with healthy skin production. Cucumbers are also super high in water, and help your skin stay hydrated. I like them with a bit of salt and lemon.
- **good oils** like olive, flaxseed, avocado, coconut, chia, hemp, evening primrose, walnut, and fish oil, as well as raw soaked/sprouted nuts and seeds, and olives themselves are vital for health and a prerequisite for lustrous skin. Healthy fats are great sources of essential fatty acids and other lipids that keep the skin soft and supple.
- **seaweeds,** such as hijiki, kombu, arame, wakame, and blue-green algae, such as spirulina and chlorella, are incredibly rich in antioxidants, vitamins, minerals, DHA and EPA omega-3 fatty acids, and iodine. There are those UV-damage-protecting antioxidants again, plus omegas for fighting acne and wrinkles by supporting the systems that manage oil production, because EPA is great for skin hydration and acne prevention.[3]

BEAUTY SMOOTHIE

You can help your skin find homeostasis—aka balance—by giving it three things: excellent nutrition to provide the building blocks (like collagen) for a beautiful glow, water to nurture and hydrate the cells, and oxygen to help your skin cells to breathe. This smoothie delivers on skin-supportive nutrition with collagen, spirulina, and plenty of antioxidants, including vitamin C, and it offers hydration from water and coconut water. So take a few deep breaths, turn the blender on, and drink up.

Serves 2

1. Add all the ingredients to a high-speed blender, putting the spinach at the bottom to ensure it blends thoroughly.

2. Blend until smooth and enjoy.

INGREDIENTS

1 cup baby spinach

½ cup coconut water

1 cup water

1 cup frozen raspberries

½ cup frozen pineapple

1 tablespoon spirulina powder

2 to 3 tablespoons collagen powder

1 tablespoon pearl powder (optional) (see page 62)

CORTISOL OVERHAUL

When it came to my skin, hormone imbalance was also a big issue, specifically my cortisol levels. Cortisol is a hormone produced by your adrenal glands. The adrenals make lots of hormones from cortisol to—you guessed it—adrenaline. These are the run-from-a-tiger hormones that saved our lives in the past, and the run-to-my-next-gig hormones that helped me maintain a modern lifestyle that was way too busy. My stressful schedule was making my adrenals work overtime; my poor hormone-makers were overtaxed and dizzy.

Everybody produces cortisol—it's what helps you wake up in the morning, which is why normal cortisol levels are usually higher in the morning and lower in the evening (my levels were reversed because of my crazy schedule). But while the right amount of cortisol is necessary, too much can be harmful, because high cortisol levels can increase heart rate, blood pressure, and blood glucose. It can also slow down the reproductive cycle and mess with digestion.

If I wanted my cortisol levels to be balanced, Monica said, I had to work on lowering my stress in the evening. I felt like she was telling me that my night job wasn't doing my face any favors.

DJing was my only income at that time, but something was going to give, and I didn't want it to be my health. If I really wanted to feel good, I was going to have to overhaul my whole lifestyle, but I was determined to keep my musical/technical skills at the forefront of whatever job I had next. I noticed that when I went to events, there would always be a DJ in the corner or on the balcony. If I could get myself into the event world, then I would free up my nights and completely change my routine while still doing what I loved.

Moving from being a nightclub DJ to an event DJ wouldn't happen overnight, but if I wanted to get my body into balance, I had to be ready to do the work. This was going to take dedication, curiosity, and patience. And as I reclaimed my evening hours, I had more space to focus on making the shifts that I wanted to make. I was able to regain my passion for cooking and working out because now I actually had time in my life to let positive things in. Things that made me feel good!

My health journey was under way. And I was hooked.

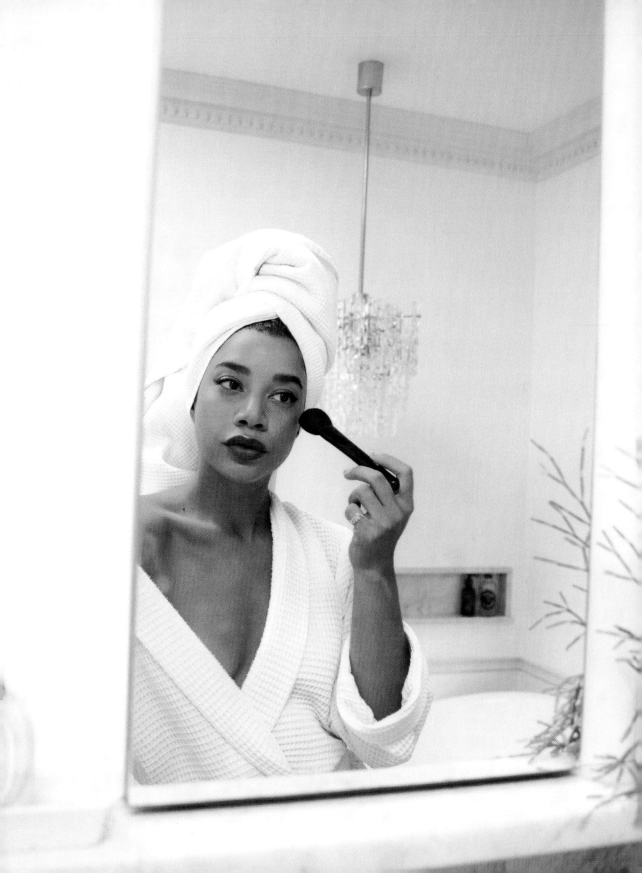

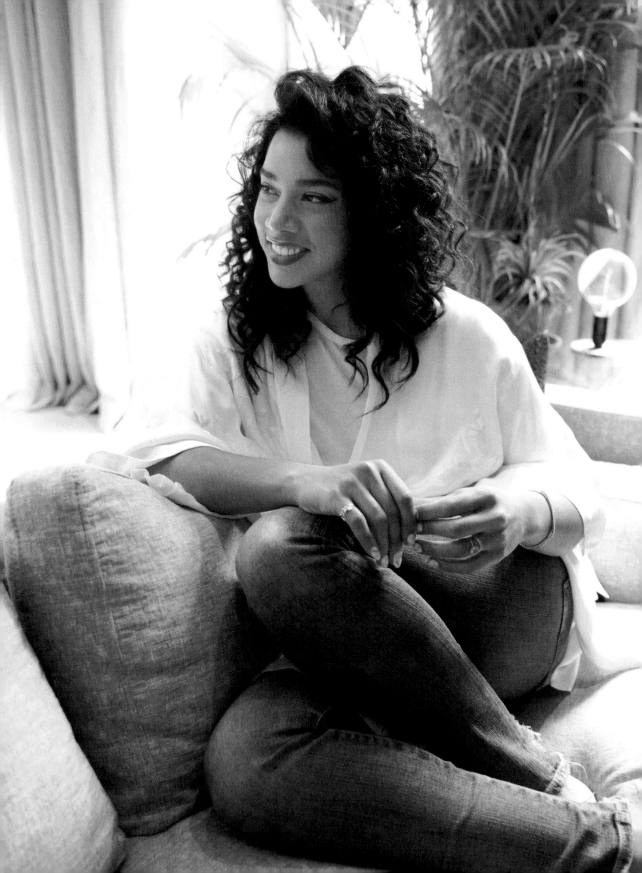

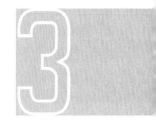

LOVE YOU, mean it

SELF-CARE STARTS WITH YOUR GUT

The road to wellness is full of potholes. Seeing positive results is the best inspiration for making healthy choices part of a consistent routine—but some old favorites still held allure for me. Like the sandwiches at the famous Katz's Deli on the Lower East Side, where I remember finding myself with my best friend at some crazy hour, even though I was working toward a healthier lifestyle. We ordered the ridiculously large pastrami sandwiches they're known for, and I ate every bite of mine. But when I got home, I was so lethargic I could barely keep my eyes open. I felt depleted, kind of sick, and just gross. I remember waking up on the couch later and thinking, "Food shouldn't make me feel this way."

At this point, I had made a lot of progress when it came to my relationship with food. I ate when I was hungry, I enjoyed my meals, and I allowed myself to eat as much as I wanted (and more, if I'm honest). But what I had been learning about health showed me that I was missing the other side of the biofeedback loop. For a long time, when the food in front of me said "Eat," I listened. When I felt like shit afterward, I didn't pause to think that perhaps my body didn't love or need the food I was feeding it. Maybe it wanted some-thing else. Maybe just like the condition of my skin was a wake-up call, all of those stomachaches and headaches, the bloating and the lethargy, were also SOS signals from my body. A series of WHAT THE FUCK ARE YOU DOING, HANNAH? texts straight from my overtaxed cells. This was a red-flag situation.

The good thing is that this time, I was ready to pay attention to the very panicked signals my body was sending.

GUT CHECK

The moment I met Tracy Piper, I felt like I was encountering Mother Earth in human form. She has beautiful energy and is so knowledgeable that I was immediately excited to learn from her. Tracy is an expert in cleansing and detoxification, a Chinese herbologist, an internal fitness doctor, and an acupuncturist. She's the author of *The Piper Protocol*, which is an amazing cleanse program. And she gives the best colonic in New York City.

Tracy opened my eyes to the importance of maintaining a healthy gut. By now you've probably heard about your microbiome, which is a collection of bacteria that hang out in your digestive tract. Over the past few years, everyone in the health and wellness community has been freaking out about the microbiome, and for good reason. Research has been connecting the health of the microbiome to the health of our gut and to our overall health and immunity.

The research on the microbiome is barely a decade old, and more studies are being published every day. But here's what we know now: You have ten times more foreign bacteria in your body than you do human cells. Those microbes help you with everything from digesting your food and extracting its nutrients to supporting the health of your immune system. They even "talk" to your brain via neurotransmitters like serotonin.[1]

But even with their powerful abilities, your microbes are fragile and very affected by the world you live in. Good bacteria can be wiped out by antibiotics sent in to kill the harmful ones, as well as by stress, personal products that are full of toxins (including beauty products!), and eating certain foods. And when you wipe out the "good" bugs, the population of bad bugs can start to overcrowd your gut. When this happens—when your microbial population is out of balance—you can get sick. You can wind up with allergies, inflammatory bowel disease, or diabetes. Imbalances in the microbiome have even been linked to cancer.[2]

Tracy opened my eyes to a whole new view of how my body worked. Literally.

CANDIDA CLAPBACK

One of Tracy's specialties is administering colonics, which is a process that uses a gentle infusion of water to clean out your colon. After I'd had a couple of colonics, Tracy said, "Your gut is really messed up because you've been on so many antibiotics and you have lots of candida in your system."

I said, "How did you know I was on antibiotics? And what is candida?"

Well, candida is yeast, and she could tell because of the contents of my colon, which we were both getting a front-row view of as she irrigated it and we watched what came out. And the situation was not pretty. As it turns out, your mouth, your skin, and your intestines are all hosts to candida, and usually you have no idea. We all have candida in our guts! But sometimes, candida becomes overgrown and starts to take over, and that's when things get funky.

Overgrown candida is super common, causing most of the fungal infections that a human body can experience.[3] Three in four women will have a yeast infection at least once. If you've ever been one of those three women, you know that yeast infections suck. It burns when you pee, your vaginal discharge becomes incredibly suspicious, and it hurts to have sex. If you get one, call your doctor to get a proper diagnosis and treatment! And keep in mind that men can get yeast infections, too. (And they can give one to you, and you can give it to them, so if you are having any of these symptoms, please, please go see a doctor and make sure it's actually a yeast infection so you can get the right treatment, because these symptoms can also point to bacterial infections or an STD.)

Yeast overgrowth can also cause some other, murkier symptoms, like general fatigue, which is what I was experiencing at the time. It can affect your digestive system, since part of the issue is that your healthy bacteria have stopped being able to moderate the amount of candida. So that was me, too.[4]

Tracy and I talked about the fact that sugar feeds yeast. I was already working on cutting out sugar out because I wanted to protect my body from inflammation, but now I had extra proof that processed sugars needed to go because all that sugar I was eating was leading to an overgrowth of yeast. Looking back now, it all makes so much sense, but at that time I didn't know how in sync, or rather out of sync, all my systems were.

My healthy bacteria needed a boost instead of a shove. Instead of supporting my system, I had been overloading it, and that was all a part of why I was feeling bad. The amount of candida in my body, I learned, was largely the result of my lifestyle: drinking too much alcohol (check), taking too many antibiotics (check), eating too many processed sugars and carbs (check), feeling super stressed all the time (check).

Tracy promised me that if I restored the health of my microbiome, my own health could be restored, too. I was in love with this woman who was telling me that I could feel good again. If she said I had to balance my gut, that was what I was going to do so I could get back to putting on my glitter eyeshadow and living my life.

EATING FOR GUT HEALTH

If you're a guinea pig like me, who always loves to try something new, you'll be scheduling a colonic for this week. If you're not so inclined (not yet, anyway), you can still improve your gut health by supporting the good bacteria that work hard to keep you healthy. Remember, all systems have yeast bacteria. It's only when the good bacteria are out of balance that the more insolent bacterial populations can thrive. When you support a healthy and balanced microbe situation, so many other things fall into place, too.

One of the best ways to support your gut is to eat foods that contain probiotics (which are your good microbes) and foods that contain prebiotics (which is food that probiotic bugs like to eat). You can also take probiotic and prebiotic supplements or digestive enzymes to help support your gut friends.

GOOD GUT FOODS

Here are a few of my favorite ways to eat for gut health.

PROBIOTIC FOODS

- **sauerkraut** is cabbage fermented in salted water. Go classic or revamped: So many indie brands are emerging that are making sauerkraut with beets and carrots, too, topped up with ginger, calendula, and all sorts of unexpected flavors.
- **kimchi** is a Korean condiment made from fermented cabbage and veggies with fish sauce. I love adding kimchi to just about every dish for some extra kick. Vegetarians, there is kimchi out there made without fish sauce—look for jars labeled accordingly.
- **pickles** are one of my favorite forms of food. These days it's easy to find a wide array of pickled veggies—not only the usual cucumbers but also pickled carrots, pickled peppers, pickled everything. For the most gut benefit, look for pickles that are fermented with salt, not those made with vinegar.
- **yogurt** made from milk contains live active cultures, but if you're dairy-free be sure to check the label of alternative yogurts to make sure they contain probiotics. Or you can make your own tummy-friendly coconut yogurt (page 102) by using probiotic capsules.
- **miso** is a fermented soybean paste. Mix it with hot water and some chopped scallions and tofu for a simple, delicious soup that will keep your gut happy.

PREBIOTIC FOODS

- **asparagus** is prebiotic-rich and easy to add to almost any dish. Eating it raw ups the benefits. I love to tuck some asparagus into an omelet.
- **bananas,** especially when slightly underripe, are rich with prebiotic fiber. I add bananas to my smoothies and slice them on top of yogurt and chia pudding.
- **onions and garlic** are the base of so many dishes, and they are also an easy

continued

continued from page 41

way to support a balanced gut!

- legumes, such as beans, are a great source of prebiotic fiber. Another good reason to go out for tacos (with black beans and rice on the side)!
- whole oats contain a kind of fiber called beta-glucan, which helps to promote gut health and has also been linked to lower cholesterol levels. Top your oatmeal with a dollop of yogurt and you've got the perfect gut-friendly breakfast!
- apples are a go-to snack for me. Luckily, they are also packed with nutrition, including polyphenol antioxidants and pectin, a type of prebiotic fiber.

THE GREAT JUICE DEBATE

You'll see loads of recipes for smoothies as you page through this book, but you won't find any juices. That's because I am not the biggest fan of juicing. If you have a day where you're not able to eat a single vegetable, I mean, sure, get your greens however you can. But too much juice on a regular basis is not a great thing. That's because juicing removes all of the fiber from the plants being juiced, and fiber is an important part of your diet. It helps you feel full and is good for digestion (and your gut bugs), so why would you remove it from your food? Plus, many juices also contain a lot of sugar—especially ones that include apple juice.

PRO SMOOTHIE

If you don't have time to eat, you can always drink your good-gut foods! This baby is loaded with gut-friendly ingredients, including banana and yogurt. Spinach gives you iron and some vitamin A for good measure.

Serves 2

1. Add all the ingredients except the probiotic capsules, if using, to a high-speed blender and blend until smooth.
2. Taste, and add stevia if needed (it will likely be sweet enough).
3. Empty the probiotic capsules, if using, into the smoothie, blend briefly to incorporate, and enjoy.

INGREDIENTS

1 cup baby spinach

¼ cup fresh basil leaves

½ cup frozen pineapple

½ cup frozen sliced strawberries

½ frozen banana

½ avocado, pitted and peeled

1 cup coconut water or water

½ cup Greek or coconut yogurt

1 tablespoon peeled and chopped fresh ginger

Stevia (optional)

2 probiotic capsules (optional)

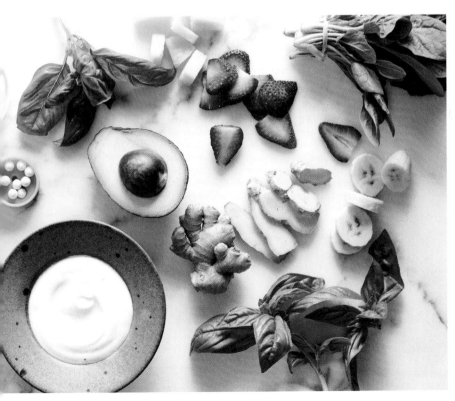

DETOX SUPPORT SMOOTHIE

INGREDIENTS

1 small beet, peeled

$\frac{1}{2}$ avocado, pitted and peeled

1 orange, peeled

$\frac{1}{2}$ cup frozen blueberries

$\frac{1}{2}$ cup frozen strawberries

1 cup steeped, cooled green tea (unsweetened)

$\frac{1}{2}$ cup water

1 tablespoon almond butter

Stevia or honey

Your liver is the detox center of your body. This heroic organ is on the front lines, taking hits for you every time you make a not-so-healthy choice.[5] It lives on the right side of your body, just under your ribs, and from command central it literally processes everything that you put in your mouth—from the greasy food to the "occasional" cigarettes to the late-night cocktails to all of the medications you've been prescribed (or are self-prescribing).

If your gut isn't doing so great, chances are neither is your liver—which has to deal with all of the toxic sludge your body can't process. This smoothie will give your poor liver some much-needed TLC. It includes beets, which are known to help boost liver function, as well as detoxifying green tea.

Serves 2

1. Blend all the ingredients except the stevia in a high-speed blender.

2. Taste, and add sweetener as needed.

3. Serve and enjoy.

do
what
feels
good

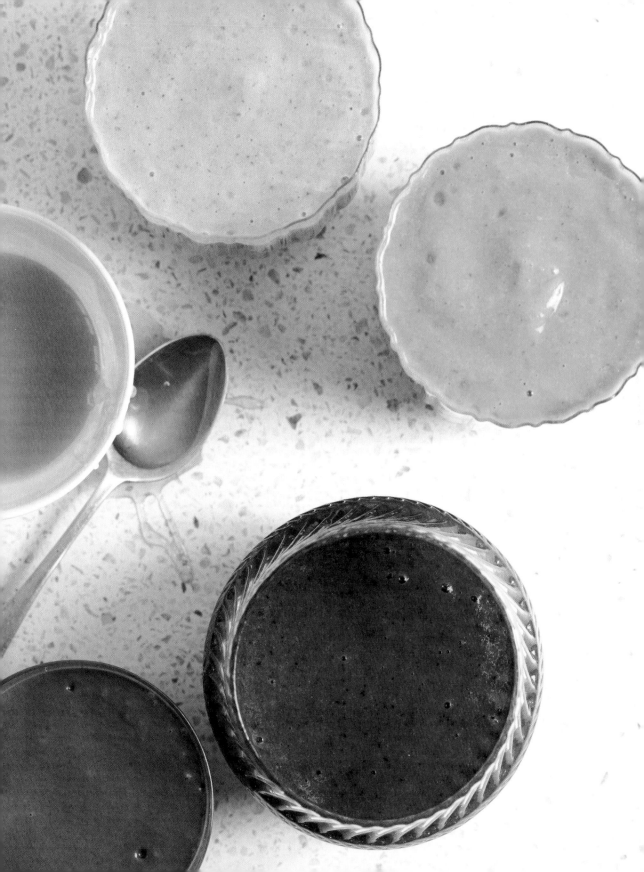

DIGESTION SMOOTHIE

INGREDIENTS

1 apple, unpeeled, chopped
(I like Honeycrisp or Gala)

2 pitted prunes

1 cup water, plus more as
needed

$\frac{1}{4}$ teaspoon ground
cinnamon

1 teaspoon honey

$\frac{1}{2}$ teaspoon pure vanilla
extract

$\frac{1}{2}$ cup plain Greek yogurt,
coconut yogurt, or almond
yogurt

1 frozen banana

1 teaspoon peeled and
grated fresh ginger

1 teaspoon peeled and
grated fresh turmeric

Your gut is the center of your health, so keeping things moving is an absolute must. If you had some weird take-out food for dinner or ate a late-night meal you regret the next day because your stomach is still feeling it, this smoothie is your friend. It's got prebiotic fiber from the apple and banana, ginger and turmeric to help settle your stomach, cinnamon to balance your blood sugar, and prunes to keep things on the regular.

Serves 2

1. Add the apple, prunes, and 1 cup of water to a high-speed blender and blend until smooth. Add more water if needed, and blend again.

2. Add the remaining ingredients and blend for 30 seconds to 1 minute.

3. Serve and enjoy.

do
what
feels
good

NEW ROUTINES, NEW RESULTS

As I started taking Tracy's advice—cutting out the sugars, paying more attention to my digestion—I felt more positive shifts taking hold. I felt a stronger connection to my body. I had more energy. I was in a better mood. I became a better girlfriend, friend, and sister. I could see and feel the difference, and so could the people who loved me, because I was so much happier (and a whole lot nicer).

When I had tried to diet in the past, I was always following somebody else's set of rules, trying to look like someone else's standard of beautiful. Then I threw all the rules out the window and did things that felt good in the moment—but weren't always great for me in the long term. Then I tried to make adjustments for the sake of my skin. But there was more at stake. I needed to understand what my body actually wanted and needed. I realized that my body would keep trying to share its wisdom through every means necessary, and I was ready to keep learning its language.

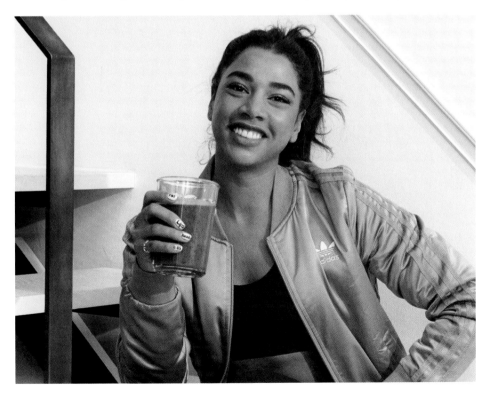

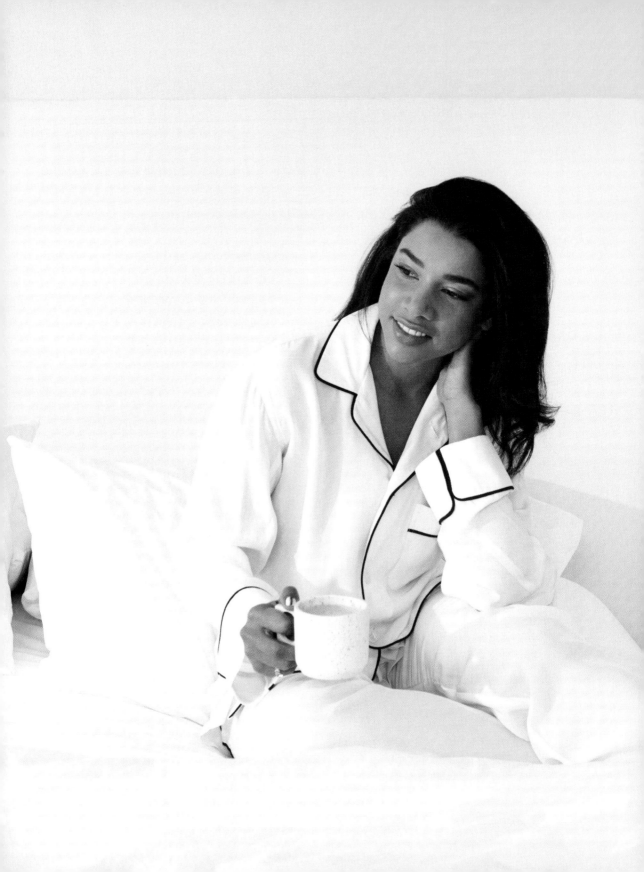

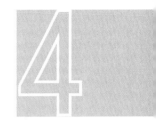

the potion PROJECT

TONICS FOR HIGHER VIBES

Every morning, after I wash my face and have a glass of water, I go downstairs and get the hot water going for a delicious tonic. What's a tonic, you ask? For me, it's a drink that includes medicinal herbs and roots that I can customize depending on how I'm feeling and what kind of support my body might need. I'm not a big coffee person, so my morning ritual includes a warm tonic that can energize me and get me ready for the day. Every evening, my nighttime ritual includes a calming tonic with soothing herbs, to help my body relax.

My tonics are a way for me to replenish. The routines give me time and space to listen to my body. I can decide what I need to feel good, right then and there. And there's something about sipping on a hot beverage that is just incredibly comforting and meditative. Every sip warms me and anchors me to the moment I'm in, giving me time to reflect and breathe and acknowledge the present.

As you already know, before I began my health journey I was living too fast, doing too much, without a supportive routine to keep me steady and balanced. For years, I had been living as an up-all-night and sleep-all-day type of chick. This whole pattern left me really depleted and stressed out. I was out of gas, running on willpower and caffeine. That was part of why my cortisol levels were so high. My body's stress hormones had been the only thing keeping me going!

The idea of "early to bed and early to rise" was totally foreign to me. Unheard of. That was someone else's life. My body was accustomed to my night-owl routine, and it took time for me to adapt to a totally different rhythm. Like most of the healthy changes I made to my lifestyle, this was NOT easy and it did NOT happen overnight. I needed support along the way, and drinking tonics became a ritual that helped me support myself as I worked hard to glow the eff up.

By creating a morning ritual, I made space for a moment of self-reflection and self-care that I could use to really set the tone for my day.

WELCOME TO THE TONIC PARTY

I first started drinking tonics when Tracy Piper gave me a morning blend that I would mix with nut milk and coconut butter to make an energizing drink. This hot latte became my morning fix. It made me feel so good that I just wanted to know more about what was in it that could have such an impact on my energy levels.

The answer was adaptogens, natural substances that help regulate our body's hormonal response to stress (of the mental and physical variety) and give our adrenal glands some much-needed support. With that knowledge in my pocket, it made perfect sense that these tonics were improving my sense of well-being.

Adaptogens come from herbs and mushrooms and roots and tree bark. Some, like ashwagandha, may be new to you, like they were new to me. Some may be old friends: ginger and turmeric are both adaptogenic roots. One of the best things about my health journey was learning about the power of adaptogens, because I'm all about giving myself an edge, especially the kind that helps my body deal with stress. As my knowledge increased and I learned more about their individual effects, I started playing with adaptogens in response to how I was feeling and what kind of support I was needing throughout the day.

Every morning, while I make my tonic, I get to take a moment to focus on me, and then I can play around with the adaptogenic profile that I put into my morning drink. How am I feeling? What do I have planned? What do I need to achieve the tasks at hand and feel good all day long? Do I have a zit? Am I getting a cold? There's a tonic for that. Or maybe I've just been going, going, going, going, so I need something that's a little bit more restorative, something that's going to be really grounding. A chill-out tonic!

I believe in the power of adaptogens to help balance our hormones and keep us feeling good in mind and body. But one of my favorite parts of my tonic routine is that it offers me a moment to take my temperature and connect with myself about

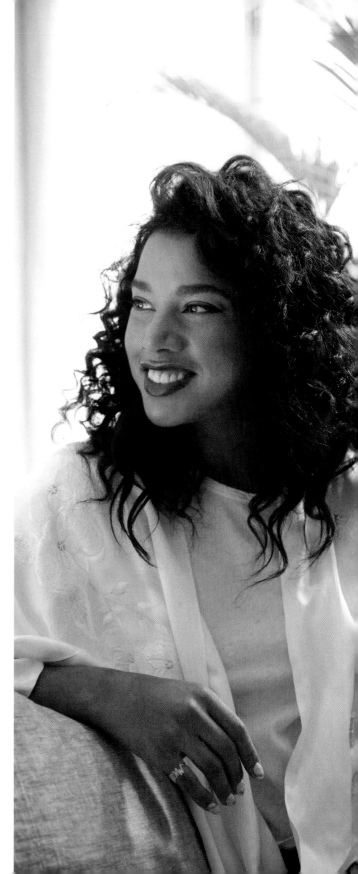

how I'm feeling. And then I can take care of myself accordingly, giving my body the tools to help keep me in balance throughout my day.

I'M FEELING SUPERSONIC (GIVE ME ADAPTOGENS AND TONIC)

You can buy adaptogens—like ashwagandha, maca, and tocos, some of my favorites—as supplements, powders, herbs, roots, and tinctures. Some of these ingredients will sound very unfamiliar, but really, drinking preparations of leaves or roots or beans mixed with hot water to feel good is nothing new. You already do it all the time. All over the world, people love a hot drink for energizing or relaxing. In Italy, they're always offering you an espresso. It's the afternoon in England, you have a serious tea session. In North Africa, where I got married, we were always greeted with mint tea. In the United States, coffee is basically served in buckets.

The thing is that we're all using these hot drinks to make us feel better, but alongside is usually heaps of sugar, which we already know isn't doing us any favors. Or those fake sweeteners usually made of chemicals. Then there's the caffeine, which is an addictive stimulant that wakes you up but can also give you the jitters. Caffeine stimulates your adrenal glands, prompting the release of cortisol.

So yes, you feel awake in the moment—but the effects of cortisol can linger well after that morning meeting you needed to power up for.[1] And if you're drinking coffee throughout the day, especially into the late afternoon or evening, you probably find that it's difficult to wind down and sleep at night.

What adaptogenic tonics offer is a gentle way to give yourself what you are really looking for when you reach for that drink—a way to feel good on your own terms. We all have changing needs and moods. Sometimes you want to feel a little sexier, sometimes you want to feel a little more relaxed. Sometimes you want to feel more focused or more energetic. Tonics are a way to nourish yourself by developing an awareness of how you feel and what you need.

Adaptogens work best when you use them regularly so that they can stay in your system and have time to work. They are powerful when taken individually—for example, maca alone can definitely energize—but they're often combined in special blends to provide an array of support. The blends that make up the tonic recipes in this chapter are designed to support hormone balance and help your body adapt to the stress of everyday life.

In the pages that follow you'll find my favorite breakfast lattes and some tonic recipes that come straight from Tracy Piper, my favorite Earth mama! These are nourishing drinks, all of them designed to support you throughout the day. I use hot water or nut milk as a base, add medicinal herbs and adaptogens to make me feel good, and finish with flavorings to make it taste good.

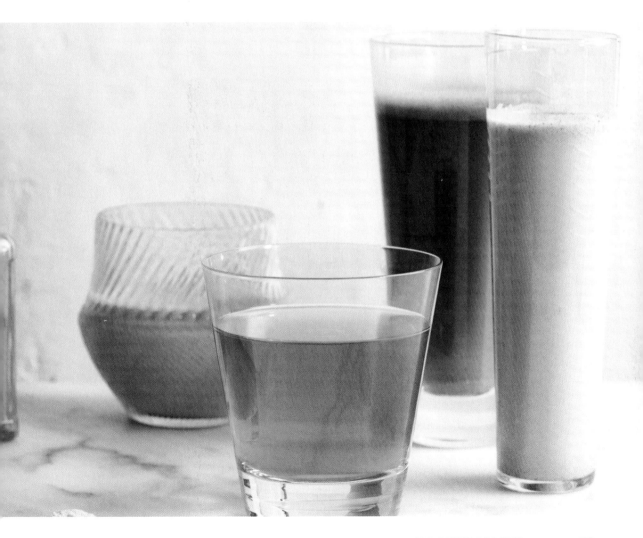

BRAIN-BOOSTING LATTE

INGREDIENTS

1 cup nondairy milk of your choice (see recipe on page 68)

1 teaspoon ghee or coconut oil

1 tablespoon MCT oil (optional)

1 shot espresso or very strong coffee

Instead of just amping yourself up with harsh caffeine, give your body what it needs to adapt to whatever will come your way. With brain-boosting MCT oil and a serving of healthy fat for satiety, this latte will help you conquer the day.

Serves 1

1. Heat the milk in a small saucepan, whisking, to make a frothy foam (or use the steamer on an espresso machine if you have one).

2. Add the ghee and the MCT oil, if using, to the milk and continue to whisk until very frothy.

3. Pour the espresso shot into a large mug and top with the milk. Serve unsweetened.

MCT OIL

MCT oil has been chatted up a lot lately because, as we have come back around to loving fats for all their health benefits, we've discovered that medium-chain triglycerides (MCTs) are especially good for the brain. MCT oil is a concentrated form of the stuff found in fats like coconut oil and butter: more than 60 percent of coconut oil is MCT, which is one of the reasons why it's so healthy. MCT is known to send all sorts of signals to your brain to help boost cognitive function, and I love it in my morning tonic because it helps me operate on another level! [2]

do
what
feels
good

TURMERIC CHAI LATTE

Turmeric has a deep yellow color when it's dried, and the fresh rhizome looks like a miniature version of ginger. Turmeric is full of curcumin, which is great for combating inflammation and boosting your immune system. This golden milk is so rich and spicy and warming, you'd never guess how healthy it is if I hadn't told you.

Serves 1

1. Heat the water, turmeric, ginger, cardamom, clove, and cinnamon stick in a small saucepan until simmering. Cover and let simmer on low for 3 to 5 minutes.

2. Remove from the heat, add the tea bag, and let steep for 4 to 5 minutes.

3. Meanwhile, heat the milk over low heat until warm, stirring occasionally.

4. Strain the spice mixture into a teacup; discard the spices. Add the milk, stir, and taste. Add honey as needed before serving.

INGREDIENTS

$\frac{1}{2}$ cup water

1 tablespoon minced fresh turmeric, ideally, or 1 teaspoon dried ground turmeric

1 teaspoon peeled and chopped fresh ginger

1 cardamom pod, or $\frac{1}{2}$ teaspoon dried ground cardamom

1 whole clove

$\frac{1}{4}$ cinnamon stick

1 black tea bag

1 cup milk of your choice (coconut and macadamia nut are great)

Honey or stevia

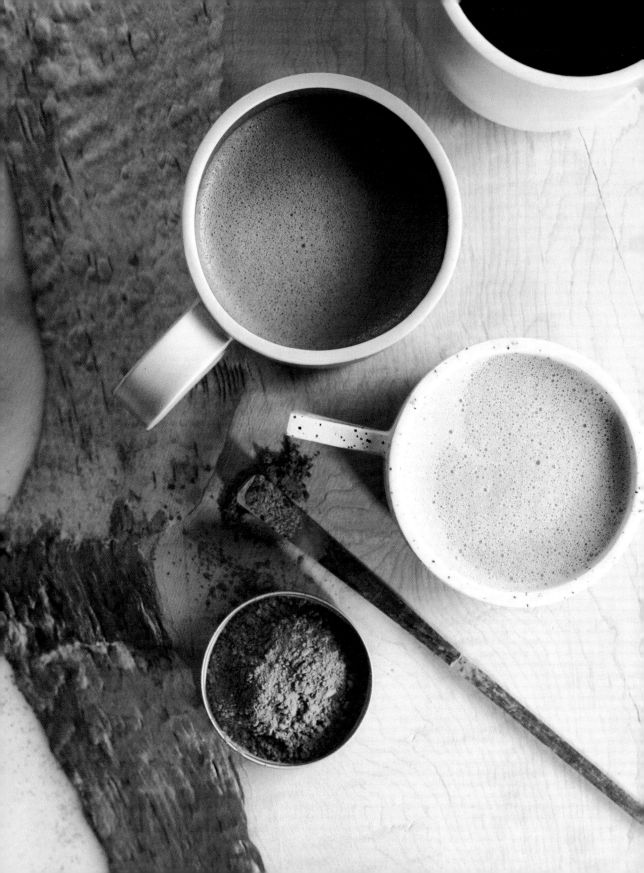

SUPERCHARGED MATCHA LATTE

Matcha is made from green tea, but the flavor is more distinctive and complex than the tea bags you steep in hot water. Matcha is made of young, delicate green tea leaves, which are ground up into a powder. It is delicious and so good for you! Matcha contains loads of anti-oxidants, necessary for skin and cellular repair, and has just the right amount of caffeine (about half of what coffee has), so it wakes you up without shoving you over an energy cliff afterward.

Serves 1

1. In a mug, whisk together the matcha powder and warm milk until frothy.

2. Whisk the ghee and MCT oil, if using, into the mixture until blended.

3. Taste, and add stevia as needed.

INGREDIENTS

1 teaspoon high-quality (ceremonial grade) powdered matcha

1 cup unsweetened coconut or cashew milk, warmed

1 teaspoon ghee or coconut oil

1 tablespoon MCT oil (optional)

Stevia

DANDELION

Dandelion—yes, the weed you used to pick in your backyard as a kid—makes an incredible tea. The roots of dandelion are really good for digestion and also help to detoxify the liver (making dandelion tea an essential if you have leaky gut—or just if you had an especially festive evening). Dandelion is a natural diuretic, which means it's also a great choice if you're dealing with bloat. I'm such a fan of dandelion root that I've created a triptych of hot drinks with it. Dandelion three ways!

DANDELION MCT COFFEE

This is my most favorite way ever to start the day. It's my go-to, my daily brew, basically my version of a pot of diner coffee that is always on and always ready to serve. If you're ever over at my place and I offer you a coffee, this is probably what I'll be making.

Serves 1

1. Heat a pot over medium-high heat and add the dandelion root and cinnamon. Toast dry, stirring occasionally, until the root becomes fragrant and golden brown.

2. Add the water and bring to a boil. Reduce the heat to a simmer and cook, covered, for 20 to 30 minutes.

3. Strain, then chill for iced coffee or serve hot.

4. When ready to drink, stir in the MCT oil.

5. Taste, and add monk fruit sweetener and coconut milk, as needed.

INGREDIENTS

1½ tablespoons dried dandelion root

1 small cinnamon stick

2 cups water

1 tablespoon MCT oil

Monk fruit sweetener (see page 60)

Coconut milk

DANDELION ROOT

You can use roasted dandelion root tea—which is widely available in stores and online—to make these drinks. If you want to try something a little different, you can also use something called Dandy Blend, which is a blend of dandelion and chicory root. It tastes like coffee when you mix it with the MCT oil. To use Dandy Blend in these recipes, swap out the tea for 1 tablespoon Dandy Blend powder. If you want a quicker morning fix, you can also use a dandelion tea bag.

CLASSIC ROASTED DANDELION TEA

INGREDIENTS

1½ tablespoons dried
dandelion root or
1 dandelion tea bag*

2 cups water

Monk fruit sweetener

Coconut milk

This beverage is similar to an English breakfast type of tea, meaning that it has the feeling of traditional black tea with milk. It's a delicious, easy, and quick way to get going in the morning.

Serves 1

1. If using dandelion root, heat a pot over medium-high heat and add the root. Toast dry, stirring occasionally, until the root becomes fragrant and golden brown. If using a tea bag, skip this step.

2. Add the water and bring to a boil.

3. Reduce the heat to a simmer and cook, covered, for 20 to 30 minutes.

4. Strain into a mug and add monk fruit sweetener and coconut milk to taste.

*If using a dandelion tea bag, steep the tea in boiling water with the cinnamon, ginger, and lemon zest for 5 minutes, then strain, add the lemon juice, and add milk and sweetener as needed.

A SWEETER SWEETENER

Monk fruit sweetener has zero calories and doesn't cause insulin spikes, which is why it's a preferred sweetener for me. I typically use a brand called Lakanto, and I like to use it in my drinks and baked goods because I enjoy the taste and love that it doesn't have the negative side effects of sugar.

do
what
feels
good

LOADED DANDELION TEA

Cinnamon and ginger add warming notes to this loaded tea, while lemon juice and zest lend a bit of sun. I drink this tea when I want something a little different that hits all my pleasure centers—flavor, energy, and a moment of calm in a busy morning.

Serves 1

1. Heat a pot over medium-high heat and add the dandelion root. Toast dry, stirring occasionally, until the root becomes fragrant and golden brown. If using a tea bag, skip this step.

2. Add the cinnamon, ginger, and lemon zest and stir to combine.

3. Add the water and bring to a boil.

4. Reduce the heat to a simmer and cook, covered, for 20 to 30 minutes.

5. Strain into a mug and add the lemon juice.

6. Taste and add coconut milk and monk fruit sweetener as needed.

*If using a dandelion tea bag, steep the tea in boiling water with the cinnamon, ginger, and lemon zest for 5 minutes, then strain, add the lemon juice, and add milk and sweetener as needed.

INGREDIENTS

$1\frac{1}{2}$ tablespoons dried dandelion root or 1 dandelion tea bag*

1 small cinnamon stick

1 teaspoon grated fresh ginger

1 large strip lemon zest

$1\frac{1}{2}$ cups water

Juice of 1 lemon

Coconut milk

Monk fruit sweetener

SKIN TONIC

INGREDIENTS

$\frac{1}{4}$ cup boiling water

1 pitted date

$\frac{3}{4}$ cup warm almond or pistachio milk

$\frac{1}{4}$ teaspoon moringa powder

$\frac{1}{4}$ teaspoon pearl powder

Of course, you know the tonic that would be my mainstay is the one that supports healthy skin. This delicious tonic gets its latte-ness from almond milk (or pistachio if you're feeling fancy), its sweetness from a date, and a hit of skin-protecting antioxidants from moringa. Moringa is a flowering plant with edible leaves that grows in Asia and Africa, and all those antioxidants help chill out the skin-harming free radicals we're exposed to on the daily. Then you've got the pearl powder, which actually comes from pearls—yes, pearls—which contain high amounts of calcium and magnesium, and which are good for your bones, teeth, and skin.[3]

Serves 1

1. Combine the boiling water and date in a high-speed blender and blend until smooth.

2. Add the remaining ingredients and blend until smooth.

3. Drink warm!

NEXT LEVEL

For even more skin support, you can also add ½ teaspoon soursop powder. Soursop comes from the guanabana tree, and extracts from the leaves are known to have antimicrobial properties that are effective against candida.[4] If you're making this with soursop, begin by whisking the soursop in hot water until well combined, then go to step 1.

do
what
feels
good

IMMUNE TONIC

Winters in New York are no joke. Everybody has a cold or the flu at some point, and if you're always on the subway or crowding into steamy little restaurants, you're going to be bombarded with germs. I like to give my system an edge by doing whatever I can to boost my immunity, starting with astragalus and schisandra berries. Astragalus is a TCM basic used for boosting energy and immunity. It's great for those times when you've got a cold or respiratory illness (or are trying to avoid one!). Then there's schisandra, which supports good circulation while it aids digestion, great for helping your body really get all the nutrients out of your food and sharing that wealth around to cells that could use some love.

Serves 1

1. Place all the ingredients in a high-speed blender and blend until smooth.

2. Taste, add stevia as needed, and serve.

*For a delicious, creamy variation, try it with macadamia milk instead of water.

2 cups water*

½ teaspoon astragalus powder

½ teaspoon schisandra berry powder

Stevia or monk fruit sweetener

STRIP-CLEAN TONIC

INGREDIENTS

4 to 6 branches of
parsley, juiced*

½ lemon, juiced*

1 celery stalk, juiced*

1 cucumber, peeled
and juiced*

1 thumb-size piece fresh
ginger, juiced*

1 green apple, juiced*

¼ teaspoon ground dried
turmeric

¼ teaspoon uva ursi powder

¼ teaspoon horsetail powder

Monk fruit sweetener

For this bright and bold detoxifying tonic, you'll be juicing some body-friendly fruit and vegetables and mixing it with turmeric, uva ursi, and horsetail powder. Turmeric works to reduce inflammation, is great for digestion, and offers solid liver support. Uva ursi is a disinfectant that supports your kidneys and bladder, and is extra good for women. Horsetail—not actually made from a horse's tail—is an herb that supports your bladder and your digestion.[5] It's all blended together with tart lemon, cleansing celery, cooling cucumber, and spicy ginger. We've included an apple for sweetness, but you can add some monk fruit sweetener if you want it a little bit sweeter.

Serves 1

1. Add the juices to a high-speed blender, along with the turmeric, uva ursi, and horsetail.

2. Blend until well combined.

3. Taste, add monk fruit sweetener as needed, and serve.

*If you don't have a juicer, you can blend the whole versions of these ingredients in a high-speed blender until smooth and strain to extract the juice.

do
what
feels
good

CHILL-OUT TONIC

This warm tonic is my go-to when I want to take it down a notch and then maybe another notch. Coconut milk is one of my favorites, and it's such a good base for this rich tonic. We've included pearl powder, ashwagandha, and shatavari. Pearl powder supplies a hit of magnesium, the mineral that is a "settle down" instruction for your body. Ashwagandha, a mainstay of Ayurvedic tradition, supports your nervous system and your adrenal glands and helps your body deal with stress. *Shatavari* means "woman who has a hundred husbands," which doesn't sound very chill at all—but this is one of the most important herbs in the Ayurvedic tradition for women's health, so I'll take it.[6]

Serves 1

INGREDIENTS

2 cups warm coconut milk

½ teaspoon pearl powder (see page 62)

½ teaspoon shatavari powder

¼ teaspoon ashwagandha powder

⅛ teaspoon ground cinnamon

Stevia or raw honey, as needed

1. Place all the ingredients except the stevia in a blender and blend until smooth and frothy.

2. Taste, and add stevia as needed; coconut milk has natural sweetness, so you may not need any.

3. Drink warm.

NEXT LEVEL

If you want to take things up a notch, you can try adding ½ teaspoon each bupleurum and dragon bone powder. Bupleurum is a Chinese herb that strengthens the liver and protects it from the harmful effects of toxins, and dragon bone powder (another incredibly named adaptogen if you ask me) is made from the fossilized bones of mastodons. A bit of a yikes for some, but it's a popular remedy in Asia that is thought to be effective for stress and sleeplessness.[7]

SLEEP-TIGHT TONIC

INGREDIENTS

1½ cups water

1 tablespoon chamomile flowers (or contents of 1 100-percent chamomile tea bag)

1 tablespoon passion flower powder (optional)

10 drops magnesium oil

5 drops food-grade lavender essential oil (YL or Doterra are two brands you can try)

Magnesium for maximum relaxation, chamomile for getting super chill, lavender for even more Zen vibes—this is the thing to sip when you really want a good night's sleep. I'm usually a very good sleeper, but sometimes there's just a lot on my mind. That's when I'll take a hot bath and follow it up with this tonic—basically a spa bath for your insides.

Serves 1

1. Heat the water to just below boiling—a light simmer is perfect.

2. Add the chamomile flowers and passion flower powder and let steep 3 to 4 minutes.

3. Strain the tea into a cup and add the magnesium and lavender oils. Stir and enjoy.

NEXT LEVEL

If you're the type who always goes for extra-strength, or you really need more sleep, you can add 1 tablespoon of passion flower powder to calm the nervous system, quiet the mind, and help you rest.

do
what
feels
good

SEX A LATTE

Kind of like a vanilla-caramel milk shake, this drink was meant to be shared and savored. Custom made for evenings of leisure and pleasure, curated for vitality and everything extra. Maca is beneficial for both women and men when it comes to sexual health. Colostrum, the milky substance that all mammals make before breast milk, increases your feelings of well-being.[8] (It comes from cows. Skip this one if you're vegan.) Then there's he shou wu, reputed to restore energy and sexual energy,[9] and lucuma, from a sweet orange Peruvian fruit, which gives the drink a hit of antioxidants and a naturally sweet caramel flavor. The MCT oil is great for your brain and helps with clarity and focus. All the better when you're with someone you really want to pay attention to.

Serves 1

1. Place all the ingredients in a blender and blend until smooth.
2. Serve topped with a little nutmeg, if desired.

INGREDIENTS

$\frac{1}{2}$ cup almond butter

$\frac{1}{4}$ teaspoon vanilla bean powder, vanilla paste, or pure vanilla extract

$\frac{1}{2}$ cup colostrum powder

$\frac{1}{2}$ teaspoon astragalus powder

$\frac{1}{4}$ teaspoon maca powder

$\frac{1}{4}$ teaspoon he shou wu powder

2 tablespoons MCT oil

2 tablespoons lucuma powder

16 ounces cashew or coconut milk

$\frac{1}{4}$ teaspoon freshly grated nutmeg

BASIC MILK

INGREDIENTS

1 cup raw nuts of your choice

2 cups water

Add-ins of your choice
(see chart on page 69)

I often incorporate nut milks into my tonics, and when I do, I try to use homemade versions. Yes, in a pinch I will definitely use store-bought varieties, but when I can I like to keep my own nut milk in the fridge. All of these milks will taste a little different depending on the nuts and add-ins you choose. I promise, once you get the hang of the process, it's super easy. And super delicious.

Makes 2 cups

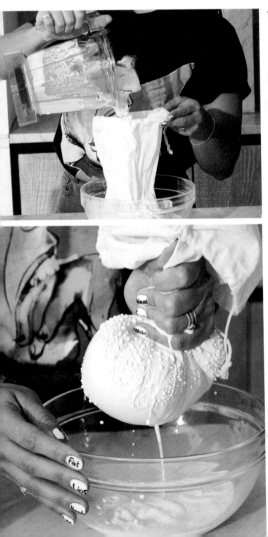

1. First you need to soak the nuts. Place the nuts in a medium bowl and pour in water to cover. Place in the refrigerator for at least 8 hours; leave for up to 3 days for a creamier milk.

2. Drain the nuts and rinse them in cool water.

3. Place the nuts in a high-speed blender and add the water.

4. Blend on the highest setting for 2 minutes (or process in a food processor for 4 to 5 minutes, pausing to scrape down the sides occasionally).

5. While the mixture is blending, line a strainer with either an opened nut milk bag (available on Amazon.com and in cooking stores) or 3 to 4 layers of cheesecloth, and place over a bowl.

6. Pour the nut mixture through the lined strainer and let drain to extract as much liquid as possible.

7. Close the bag or wrap up the ends of the cheesecloth and squeeze/press the mixture to extract as much remaining liquid as possible.

8. Taste the milk, and blend with add-ins of your choice.

9. Store the nut milk in a sealed container in the fridge for up to 3 days, or freeze for 2 to 3 months.

DIY MILK

BASE	POSSIBLE ADD-INS	NOTES
ALMOND	Stevia or monk fruit sweetener, cinnamon stick	If adding cinnamon, add the stick during the soaking process, but only for the last 4–8 hours, unless you like a very strong cinnamon flavor. Remove before blending.
HAZELNUT	Maple or monk fruit sweetener, vanilla bean	If adding vanilla, split the bean and add it for the soaking process. You may find it adds a sweet enough essence that you don't need sweetener. Remove before blending.
COCONUT	Ginger root (best unsweetened)	If using shredded, unsweetened coconut, use 2–3 cups. If using chunks of coconut meat, use 3–4 cups, and reduce the water by half. If adding ginger, add for the last 3 hours of the soak, and start small — it's a strong flavor.
CASHEW	Honey or stevia, turmeric, cinnamon stick	If adding cinnamon, add the stick during the soaking process, but only for the last 4–8 hours, unless you like a very strong cinnamon flavor. Remove before blending. If adding turmeric, grate a root into the mixture, leave in for blending and straining (but be prepared to have your cloth stained).
MACADAMIA	Best plain, unsweetened	Benefits from a longer soak (24–48 hours) and makes a very creamy, neutral-tasting milk that's great in coffee.
OAT	Cinnamon, vanilla bean, maple or monk fruit sweetener	For a richer, deeper flavor, try toasting the oats in a dry pan before soaking. Make sure to remove cinnamon or vanilla bean before blending.
PECAN OR WALNUT	Maple or monk fruit sweetener, allspice	Try toasting the nuts before soaking for a very rich, nutty flavor. If adding whole allspice berries, only add for last 4–8 hours, and remove before blending.
BRAZIL NUT	Stevia	Benefits from a longer soak (24–48 hours) and makes a very creamy, neutral-tasting milk that's great in coffee.
HEMP	Stevia, $\frac{1}{4}$ teaspoon of sea salt	For this one, grind the seeds with water and salt right away — no soaking or straining needed!

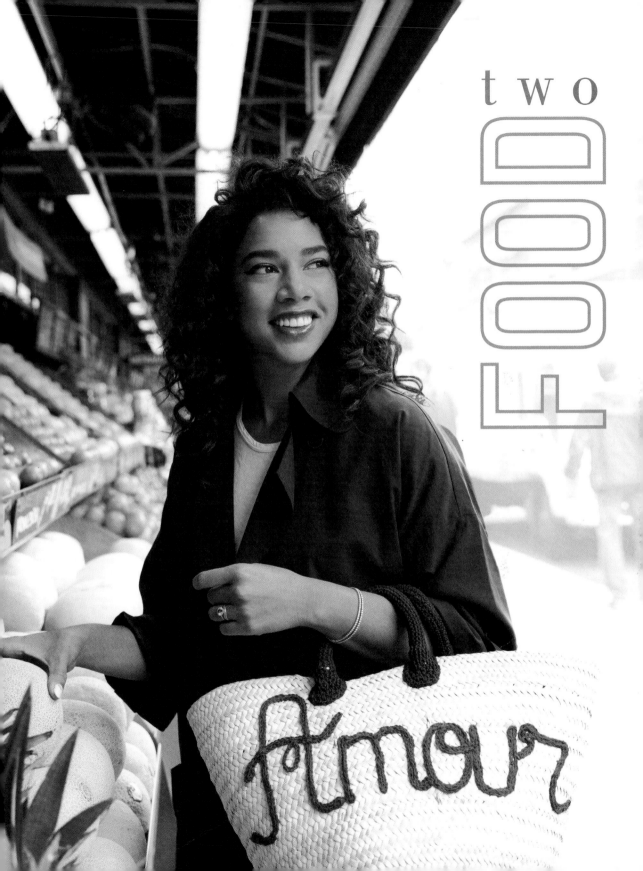

two

FOOD

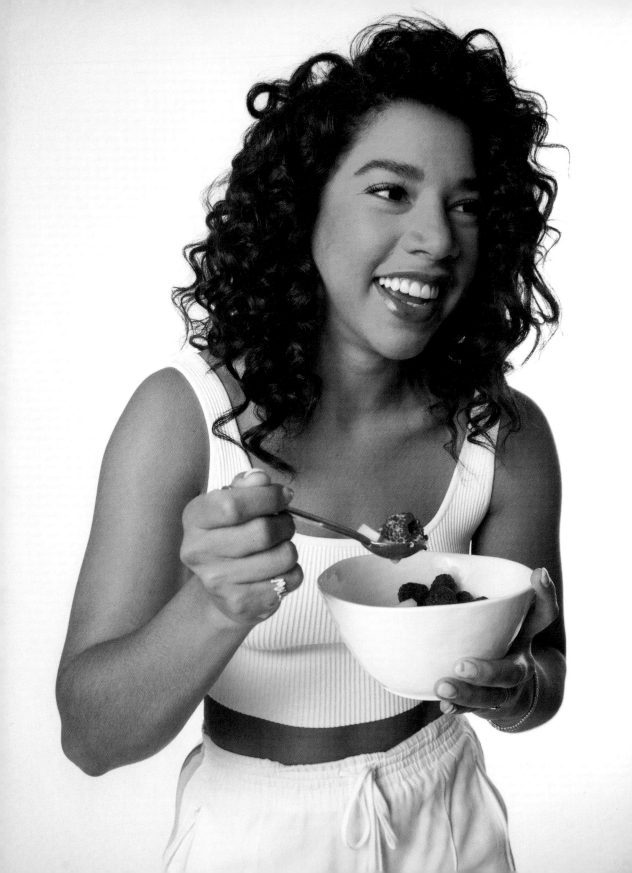

everything's better
WITH ALMOND BUTTER

EAT WHAT FEELS GOOD

I grew up in a vegetarian household (my mom was a true child of the '70s). I had my first burger at age seventeen. Seventeen!!! It was a total game-changer. After I realized how many other flavors I'd never experienced, I devoted myself to expanding my palate. I wanted to explore all the foods, and the more I sampled and tasted, the more adventurous I became. And I still am. At home or in restaurants, I just want to try absolutely everything.

As a little girl I loved being in the kitchen. I can remember my mom having dinner parties and she always hired the same caterer, Ms. Norma Jean. Ms. Norma would have me asking the guests what they wanted to drink, and sometimes if I was lucky I could bring out the appetizers and explain what each dish was. I was always in and around the kitchen, so wanting to be a skilled at-home chef has always been a part of my DNA. I'm not saying I'm a professional by any stretch, but I do love cooking and I love to have fun with food. I love getting my hands dirty and trying out new flavors. I love the rhythm of chopping vegetables and the neat precision of baking—I find it relaxing and therapeutic.

Most of the time I keep things simple: I whip up dishes with a handful of ingredients I have in the fridge and add my favorite flavors—garlic or turmeric, paprika or za'atar. I rarely follow a recipe to the letter—I like to tweak it to my tastes. To me, more cinnamon, less garlic, and "oops I burnt that" are all a part of the experience. I start with a recipe or an idea or a craving. Then I build on the basics to create something that really speaks to me, that feels like what I need at the moment. Of course, it doesn't always work out the way I want it to, but I think trying new techniques helps me grow as a cook, and trying new foods and flavor combinations helps me grow my palate.

A lot of the time I'm just cooking for one (me) or two (plus Brendan), but I also really love cooking for a crowd. I used to have a group of friends in college who would take turns hosting potluck dinners at each of our houses, and I loved the ritual of sharing a communal meal. I always say #feedyourfriends because it's so rewarding to nurture the people you love with nourishing food. And food prepared with love tastes better! I truly believe that the positive energy you put into your food helps make other people feel good. Which, of course, makes you feel good.

For myself and for others, I focus on cooking food that is simple, healthy, and delicious, so those are the kinds of recipes you'll find here. Simple to make. Super fun to eat and share. Nourishing for your body and mind. I try not to pay too much attention to specialized eating styles and

> It's so rewarding to nurture the people you love with nourishing food.

diets. Trust me, I've tried them all. Now I just choose what feels good for my body. No two people have the exact same nutritional needs, so it's kind of crazy to think that there's one diet out there that's the right fit for all of us.

Food trends come and go. There's always going to be some cool superfood that everyone is eating, and there's always going to be a new "plan" that people swear by: vegan, paleo, keto, gluten-free—the list goes on. I think there are benefits to following a routine, and I also think there's a lot of value in many of these eating styles. But for me, doing something that feels strict and depriving doesn't work because it doesn't feel good. Moderation and flexibility are critically important to me.

In addition to being flexible and allowing myself all things in moderation, my personal key word when it comes to nutrition is *balance*. Eating a wide array of vegetables helps me keep my immune system strong, my gut bacteria happy, and my digestion moving. Eating protein with every meal helps me maintain my muscle density and tone. Healthy fats are great for my skin and help me feel satisfied and keep me from chowing down on stuff I'll regret later.

That's why the recipes in this book focus on vegetables and protein and fat and complex carbohydrates. There's not much dairy because a little bit of dairy goes a long way for me. Too much dairy makes me feel bloated; bloated doesn't feel good. Besides, there are so many creamy alternatives like nut spreads and nut milks, I don't often need to use dairy. I do include some recipes with yogurt because fermented dairy is easier on the system and comes with all those useful probiotics.

You'll also notice that there aren't any wheat-based recipes in this book. Gluten gives me a bellyache; again, not good, so although pastas are delicious, as is pizza, I've found some fabulous alternatives to these traditional staples—like lentil pasta and cauliflower pizza crust. I avoid refined sugars as well, so you won't find any here—even in the dessert section. And no artificial sweeteners in these recipes either: all those chemicals make me break out, and anyway I prefer real foods to fake ones. The more you get used to listening to your body, the more you'll be able to give it what it really wants and needs.

To me, balance means nurturing myself in every way, including enjoying (vegan) cheesecake and some of the best cocktails this side of whatever bespoke cocktail bar you frequent. If it makes you truly feel good, then it's the kind of indulgence that has a place in a balanced eating style.

BODEGA TO GO

Some days, we have the time to take care of ourselves in all our favorite ways. We exercise, we do our whole skincare routine, we make ourselves beautiful meals. Other days we don't even have time to take a shower let alone moisturize our shins, and we have zero time for meal preparation. Whether you're a businesswoman, a mother, a teacher, a student, a freelancer, or still figuring it out (or all of the above!), these days happen. Instead of freaking out, I like to arm myself with healthy snacks so that when I'm in an airport with no good choices or stuck in back-to-back meetings, I can reach in my bag and pull out a quick fix of healthiness. I get to savor the snack and the fact that I'm doing something to take care of myself. Without those treats on hand, I'm much more likely to be reaching for whatever food happens to be in front of me. Because let's face it, everything looks delicious when you're hungry, and it's that exact moment that you start making excuses like "There's nothing else around!!!" and wondering "Why is this candy staring me in the face?!?" Here are some of my fave snacks on the go:

- Almond butter packets
- Bars like 22 Days Nutrition Bars, Bulletproof Bars, NuGo Slim Bars, No Cow Bars (probably my favorite), and Kind Bars
- Dried chickpea snacks
- Seaweed snacks
- Easy-to-pack whole fruit like apples or pears
- Raw or roasted nuts
- Sometimes I'll even put a container of yogurt in my bag!

FOOD IS LIKE SEX

A wise woman once told me that eating a meal is like having sex. If you're not present and in the moment, it's not going to work. You have to be engaged, focused, and willing to participate without distractions. Eating is a sensory act. The scent of food makes it taste better, and smelling food prompts your body to create the enzymes (via your saliva) that help it digest your food. The act of eating should be

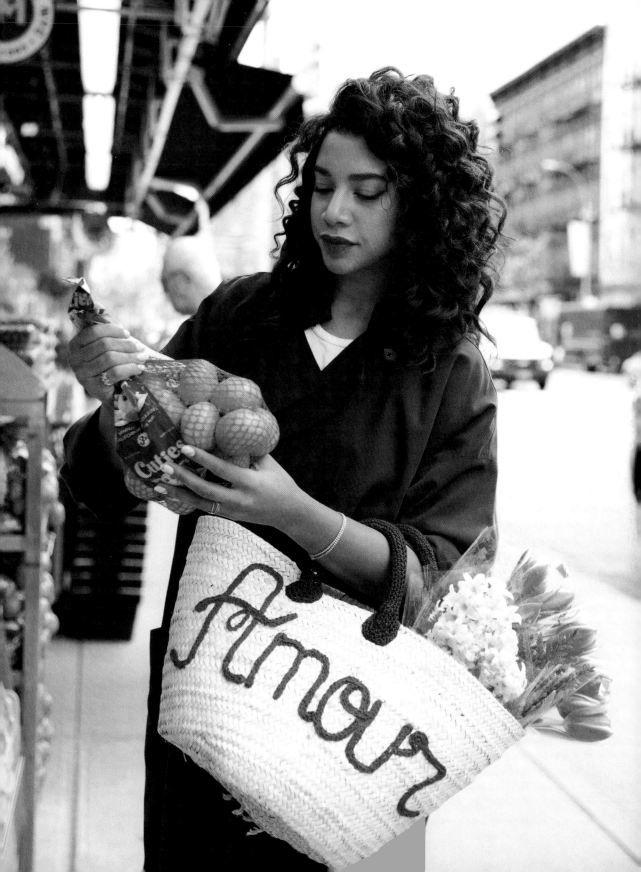

sensual and pleasurable—it should make you feel fucking awesome.

In my mind eating healthfully is the ultimate in hedonism. The easiest way to be consistent about my nutrition is to be indulgent in all the right places: If I'm loving it, I'll keep doing it. That's why I focus on bringing the joy back to eating. Remember, hunger is your friend: It is a message from your body that you need some fuel. There should be no guilt in giving energy to your body!! Mindful cooking and mindful eating are where I want to be. You have to know how food makes you feel to know what you should be eating. When's the last time you paused to check in with your body when you were eating, or afterward? When you pay attention to the way food makes you feel, you can learn a lot about what your body needs. Because we're all different.

We all have different di-

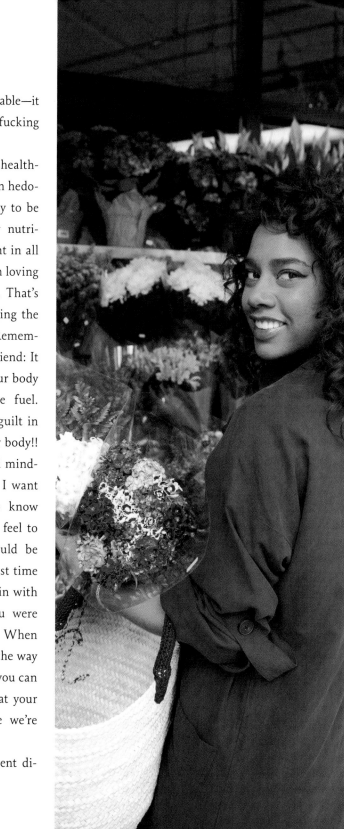

gestion. Your body might love ice cream, but mine definitely does not. I love almond and coconut flours, and you might be just fine with wheat. What we like when it comes to our food is about the taste, of course, but also about so much more. When we slow down and really savor our food, we can notice the way it makes us feel in our bodies: The comfort that comes from spooning your way through a warm bowl of soup laced with spices. The satisfaction you enjoy after savoring a sweet indulgence. That pop of energy and lightness you get after eating a salad of fresh leafy greens. Or conversely, waking up in the middle of the night with a crazy stomachache and realizing that the *cacio e pepe* is just not agreeing with you, no matter how cheesy and delicious it was in the moment.

In order to notice any of these experiences, you have to pay attention to your body's signals.

That's part of why I like to try out different ways of eating—to see how it makes me feel, to get out of ingrained patterns and be more intentional. I like to be in-

> When you pay attention to the way food makes you feel, you can learn a lot about what your body needs. Because we're all different.

tuitive when I cook, and I like to be intuitive about how I eat. This requires some practice and taking some risks, but if you get into the rhythm of physical awareness, starting in the morning, continuing all through the day, you'll find that you won't be able to stop. Before you put anything into your body, consider what it is and why you want it. How hungry are you? What are you in the mood for? What foods have been missing from your day? You may have already had fresh greens at lunch, or maybe you need to add some to your dinner. You may have had an extra-big breakfast and now you want a lighter lunch. I don't want to eat food just because it's in front of me. I want to eat it because I need it, because I want it, and because it will make me feel good.

That's true of desserts, too. If you've been eating beautifully all day and you want some chocolate cherry coconut-based ice cream (page 233), by all means, dig in. Scoop it into a lovely little bowl. Set it at the table. Sit down in front of it—no standing hunched over a counter eating as if you're trying to get away with a crime! It's something you're doing for yourself, to make yourself *feel good*.

You know what does not feel good? Regret. Self-doubt. Also, eating too much ice cream doesn't actually feel good. Savoring food crafted with care, mindfully enjoying what's on your plate, having one portion instead of five—things like these are what makes me love my food. So get back to your chocolate cherry coco ice cream. Dip in your spoon. Feel the way it hits your mouth—that cold burst, the icy spoon, the rich chocolate, the essence of cherry coming through to brighten it all up.

If it's worth eating, it should be worth enjoying.

PICK IT LIKE YOU MEAN IT

Healthy eating starts with healthy pantry management—you want to keep what works, get rid of what doesn't work, and always try new stuff for variety. Personally, I try to keep shelf-stable nut milks and dried grains around; cans of beans for a last-minute salad add-in; my fruit bowl full of oranges and lemons and avocados; my produce drawer full of herbs and leafy greens and colorful vegetables so that I can have what I want when I want it.

Keeping my pantry well stocked always feels like a good strategy so that when I want to make dinner on a busy weeknight or a rainy Sunday, I don't have to drag my butt to the grocery store. (Seriously, is there anything worse than going to the grocery store at 5:00 p.m. along with everyone else in the world to get the two items you need? And then standing in an "express" line for ten minutes to purchase those two items? Ahhhh, I could literally lose my mind just thinking about it.)

When I go to the grocery store without a list, I find myself wandering the aisles and putting things in my basket that I don't actually need. So whenever possible, I try to keep a running list on my phone and focus on picking up those items, with a little bit of room for experimentation just in case some glorious fruit or veggie catches my eye. I try to go to the grocery store once a week and the farmers' market once a week; that way I always have fresh produce that's crisp

> If it's worth eating, it should be worth enjoying.

do
what
feels
good

and delicious. If I overbuy, that produce doesn't look so great midweek.

I'm lucky enough to live in a city with an abundance of farmers' markets on different days of the week so I can pick up what I need whenever. If the farmers' markets closest to you are only open on the weekend, maybe you pick up your produce for the week there and grab any additional necessities at the grocery store. After all, the produce at the farmers' market is usually local, which means it will last longer (it hasn't been shipped across the country or the ocean and sat on trucks for days). Meal prepping is always a good idea, too, especially if you know you have a busy week ahead.

Like most other kinds of shopping, food shopping can be fun—you get to select for yourself the ripest fruits, the most beautiful veggies, the most amazing-smelling bread. But given the ever-changing state of our food system, food shopping can also be confusing and stressful.

Here are a few of the strategies I use to put the "shop" back in grocery shopping— including outsourcing when necessary.

- **all about those labels:** There's a lot of information on a food label, all of it important depending on what your needs are. I'm always on the lookout for added sugars and preservatives, because those things do not jibe with me. For you it may be sodium or gluten. I always read a food label thoroughly before trying a new product to make sure there are no surprises.

- **fresh over frozen:** I avoid processed frozen foods, though the occasional cauliflower pizza crust in a box can sometimes be an easy quick fix for dinner. Frozen organic berries are also an easy grab if the farmers' market is sold out of fresh ones.

- **nuts and fruits for the win:** I skip the processed snack sections in favor of nuts and fruits—just as portable as processed snacks but way, way better for you.

- **on the couch and on the road:** I buy for home and for travel: A dropper of stevia for smoothies on the go or at home. A jar of almond butter for my pantry, and almond butter in single-serving tubes for a quick snack between meetings.

- **delivery systems:** Sometimes there just isn't time to hit the market. Luckily, there are so many people just waiting for you to ask them to help you out here. Local grocery stores sometimes offer delivery; bulk rice or frozen coconut meat or specialty items like adaptogens can be ordered online. Especially in cities, there are so many brands and apps that will deliver fresh foods to your door if you just click "buy."

ORGANIC ORACLE

Like most people these days, I make an effort to buy organic whenever possible. I don't need to list all of the reasons why organic food is important to your health—you can read about that in a million other books. But I do try to cook with organic ingredients. Instead of writing "organic" next to every ingredient in the recipes, let me just make this blanket statement: Whenever possible, try to buy organic.

I know that this can sometimes be an additional expense or make for a less convenient errand. I get that those are real considerations, and you have to do what's right for your budget and lifestyle. But I would suggest that your health is also an important consideration. You deserve high-quality nutrition that makes you feel good. And more often than not, that nutrition comes from organic produce and responsibly raised proteins. If you cannot get organic produce, I do suggest finding your local farmers and buying your produce from them. Sometimes knowing

THE DIRTY DOZEN

The produce on this list has a dirty little secret: loads of pesticides.

It is actually a baker's dozen, because we've included hot peppers. I love spice, and capsaicin is really great for you, but I'll be loving it from an organic source only, since 75 percent of the conventional hot peppers the Environmental Working Group (EWG) tested showed up with pesticide residue.

For the stuff listed here, buy organic, not conventional.

Strawberries	Peaches	Celery
Spinach	Cherries	Potatoes
Nectarines	Pears	Sweet bell peppers
Apples	Tomatoes	Hot peppers
Grapes		

your local, small-scale food sources is even more powerful than an "organic" label.

The good news is that it is easier than ever to buy organic these days. If you see "organic" on a food label, you know that the Department of Agriculture is telling you that this food was not genetically engineered, does not have synthetic chemicals or fertilizers on it, and has not been exposed to radiation or sewage sludge.[1] And sewage-sludge-free is a health craze I can get behind.

And what about GMOs—genetically modified organisms? Yikes and double yikes. Modified seeds become crops that can do stuff they didn't do naturally, like resist certain insects or stand up to weed killers. Proponents point to crops that can survive droughts or flooding, which could help with starvation around the world. But GMOs are changing everything about how farmers farm. It used to be that farmers would save seeds to use from one season to another—and by "used to be," I mean for thousands of years. But with GMOs, farmers need to buy seeds every year. Once a company creates a seed that they own the rights to, farmers can't use it unless they

THE CLEAN FIFTEEN

In some cases, conventional isn't the worst; those are ones that are listed in the clean fifteen. When avocados were checked, only 1 in 360 had pesticide residue, while 86 percent of cabbage was cool. Broccoli samples were 70 percent clear, and 90 percent of conventional pineapples were just perf.

For the following fruits and vegetables, you can aim for organic, but you can still feel comfortable buying conventional if that is what's available or fits your budget.

Avocados	Asparagus	Kiwifruit
Pineapples	Mangoes	Cantaloupes
Cabbages	Eggplants	Cauliflower
Onions	Honeydew melons	Broccoli
Sweet peas, frozen	Sweet corn	Papayas

pay for it, which is a major threat to family farms around the world.

As far as your health, the safety of GMOs for humans isn't known yet. If this isn't your thing—and it isn't mine—it's another reason to buy organic produce.[2]

This is all a part of why buying organic feels responsible, not to mention supporting farmers with solid ethics who are working hard to deliver quality produce. But buying organic can also start to feel expensive. The EWG is one trustworthy source of divina-tion for food that has the least amount of pesticides even if it isn't designated as organic. Every year, the EWG puts out a list of the dirtiest and cleanest fruits and vegetables around so that you can navigate the conventional/organic situation.

In some cases, it turns out, conventional is okay. In other cases, you want to only buy organic and avoid conventional like it has neurotoxins (which it actually, really, truly might—and how f'ing nasty and scary is that?).

GENETICALLY MODIFIED THREE

GMO ALERT!! (Sirens blazing.) Some of the produce that you buy in the United States comes from seeds that are genetically modified.

The following three can be GMO if you buy conventional:

Sweet corn   Summer squash

Papayas

You should also be aware that, soon, apples and potatoes that are genetically modified may be showing up in stores.

WHAT'S IN A LABEL?: ANIMAL PROTEIN

When choosing animal protein, it's important to record labels. Conventional meats can contain hormones and antibiotics that have nasty side effects for humans. Some cows and chickens live in deplorable conditions, some get to go outside occasionally, and some get to go outside and eat organic grasses. Looking at labels is key but can be confusing: The fact is that not all of these claims made on labels are mandated or checked into by a single source, and the definitions can be broad. With that in mind, here's a quick breakdown of the latest terminology.

organic: When it comes to animal products, *organic* means that the animal was given organic feed, no antibiotics, and no growth hormones. It was allowed to go outside and walk around on organic land sometimes. Organic chickens have more omega-3 fatty acids and less incidence of salmonella and are not fed GMOs.[3]

grass-fed cattle: Grass-fed animals are given mother's milk and grass from birth. Grass-fed meat may be lower in fat; have more omega-3 fatty acids, which are good for your heart; and more vitamins.

free-range birds: With no cage, hens can walk around, and get to go outside sometimes. This doesn't necessarily mean that the hens are really roaming free, in case you're imagining an idyllic hilltop in the sun.

As far as chicken goes, free-range is a lot better than conventionally raised, which has been linked to health concerns, including polycystic ovary syndrome, because of the hormones. And the eggs can be better for you, with more omega-3s and vitamin E and less cholesterol.[4] But this label is also misleading because there isn't a clear standard and farms aren't inspected.

pasture-raised: For meat, dairy, poultry, and eggs, this label means the animals were raised on an organically managed pasture with supplemental organic grains.

farm-raised salmon: In this case, the "farm" means some kind of aquatic tank; two-thirds of the salmon in the United States is farm-raised. This kind of salmon can have more omega-3 fats than their wild cousins, but some studies show the quality of omega-3 is not as high. Plus, they contain more pollutants and contaminants (such as antibiotics) than wild-caught fish.

wild-caught salmon: This means the fish was caught in the ocean—but potentially caught in a very polluted ocean. The benefit of wild-caught salmon is that it can be lower in fat and higher in protein because of the fish's active lifestyle (maybe there should be a "swimming upstream" fitness trend), and the fish eat a natural diet and are not fed antibiotics.[5]

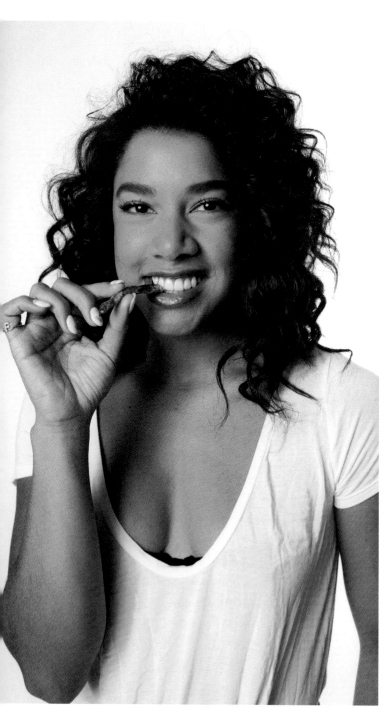

PANTRY STOCKIST, LEFTOVER QUEEN

I'm all about a pantry full of possibilities and a fridge full of leftovers. That's because I love to eat. And if I want to eat stuff I love, I need to make sure it's accessible because I don't believe that hunger is suppressible.

Honesty moment: I think about food a lot. Sometimes I feel like I'm thinking about food all day. I mean, I guess I kind of am. I'm looking up recipes and writing out shopping lists and visualizing what I'm going to make later that day or the next day or that weekend.

Cooking a good meal with precision or on the fly requires having food on hand to mess around with. If you're planning a menu for yourself or an event and you want to make something specific, you have to know what you want to make, have a recipe or some idea of how to make it, and have the right ingredients. If you encounter a mealtime where you haven't had a chance to plan, but your pantry is loaded, you'll have more options for eating simply, cooking creatively, or finding a recipe that will work with what you have on hand. With a stocked pantry you're set whether you know what you want to make or not.

What follows isn't necessarily a list of ingredients that I always have in my pantry at all times; I'm always buying different things, and I shop based on what I'm craving in the moment and in the season, or on the meals I'm planning. What these foods represent are the kinds of things I fill my basket with at the market and my fruit bowls with at home. It's a gathering of what I lean toward when I'm packing my pantry and my refrigerator, as well as the kinds of things I might make when I get home.

Stocking up makes me feel good on all the levels. First, what a joyous feeling it is to come downstairs in the morning, or come home in the evening, and know that there is all this goodness just waiting for me. It's this sensation of abundance, like the world is full of what I need and it's there for the taking. And practically, it helps make my meal prep a lot easier. I can throw together a quick bite without cooking, just by assembling ingredients in a bowl, like slicing a perfectly ripe avocado and sprinkling on some seasonings—no recipe required.

Truth: Warming up leftovers or even making a quick stir-fry takes less time than delivery and is way more satisfying.

And the stronger your pantry game is, the more you can make yourself nutrient-rich meals, usually lending themselves to more leftovers for later. And leftovers, my friends, make you a ruler of your domain. Because at the end of a busy day, when your home kingdom has a stocked pantry and fridge and you can choose to eat homemade foods instead of ordering in less-healthy foods just because you're starving—well, how good does that feel? I'll tell you. It feels really fucking good.

VEGETABLES

leafy greens: My go-to greens are spinach and arugula. I also love endive, Bibb lettuce, and baby kale. I like to have at least two kinds of greens around so I can assemble a salad at a moment's notice. Spinach and kale are equally good cooked or raw; arugula is a great green for a salad and much better consumed raw.

zucchini: I use a peeler to create noodles or make Zucchini Nests (page 111).

cucumbers: Love these cut lengthwise and topped with a sprinkle of sea salt and lemon and red chile flakes! Also amazing with a little sesame oil and sesame seeds.

beets: Raw or roasted, in salads or smoothies or pureed into a dip!

asparagus: Delicious fresh or tossed with oil and salt and roasted; either way a little lemon zest is a must.

long beans/green beans: Possibly the easiest, best crunchy snack and a great veggie to dip with or to add to a salad.

avocado: My favorite food. Avocado on everything, please. Like Avocado Egg Cups (page 110), Avocado–Smoked Salmon Toast (page 122), and "Avo-mango-rita" (yes, I said it—page 218).

radishes: I snack on whole radishes with hummus or nut spread or with just a little salt.

mushrooms: Good for adding some extra umami flavor to any dish. They pair well with eggs, too, like in my Herb and 'Shrooms Frittata (page 114).

broccoli: The perfect add-in to any salad.

It also adds the green to one of my favorite broths, The Supergreen (page 130).

cauliflower: I love cauliflower in so many versions—as a pizza crust (page 180), sliced into hearty steaks (page 179), or served as "rice" in a bowl or stir-fry.

sea vegetables: I like to keep dried seaweed on hand and sprinkle it onto salads and soups.

eggplant: For Eggplant Parm (page 196)—of course.

celery: I add it to my smoothies and love to dip a stalk into almond butter for a crunchy mouthful.

leeks: They pair well with just about anything, especially a nice piece of fish. And when roasted, they melt in your mouth!

brussels sprouts: Love, love, love me some Brussels, either halved and roasted or shaved thin for a salad with a lemony dressing.

cabbage: Slice finely and add to salads for some extra crunch.

ANIMAL PROTEIN

lean sliced turkey (nitrogen-free, from a good deli!): This is a go-to protein source for me. Turkey and cucumber with extra mustard and pepper is one of my favorite superfast snacks.

salmon: I prefer wild-caught, and I try to eat it once a week. If you're in a salmon rut, change things up with my Salt-Cured Salmon recipe (page 184)!

chicken: Brothed or braised, pastured chicken is an easy option for a weeknight meal.

eggs: Omega-3 eggs are perfect for a hit of protein in a hurry; when I'm feeling leisurely, they still serve nicely, especially in my Baked Eggs in Hash (page 119).

NUTS, SEEDS, AND BEANS

all the nuts: Pistachios, almonds, cashews, walnuts, pecans, macadamias—I use nuts for my milks, salads, desserts, and roasted with spices to snack on all day long.

quinoa: This seed cooks up like a grain, is so versatile, and is packed with protein. It's a perfect base for veggie bowls.

chia seeds: These seeds are packed with omega-3 and fiber goodness, and Basic Chia Pudding (page 99) couldn't be easier to whip up. You will find my favorite variations on pages 99 and 101.

beans: Black beans, white beans, adzuki beans, chickpeas. Keep some cans around to add healthy complex carbs and proteins to your lunch salad.

powdered almond butter: My obsession! It's amazing with apples, celery, carrots, a piece of dark chocolate, and a pinch of salt—just about anything, really.

tahini: This sesame butter is so good in salad dressings (and in hummus!).

coconut butter: I'll eat a spoonful straight up, add it to a smoothie for some healthy fat, or use it in my Blue Majik Beauty Butter (page 147).

HERBS AND SPICES

ginger: This root is a must for sick days and for my favorite Turmeric Chai Latte (page 55).

basil: Can't make a Margherita Frittata without it (page 115).

cinnamon: What isn't made better by a sprinkle of cinnamon? I add it to yogurt, chia pudding, smoothies, and tonics, and I use it in my baking.

cayenne: I like to add a little cayenne to any dish (or drink) that needs some heat.

I use it in my Cauliflower Steaks (page 179) as well as my Extra-Hot Toddy (page 212).

rosemary: Love the smell and flavor of this woodsy herb. It's great with chicken, roasted vegetables, or in my Bacon, Onion, and Potato Hash (page 118).

nutmeg: Everyone's favorite fall spice is delicious in so many dishes, from Protein Pancakes (page 107) to, yes, Pumpkin Pie X Coconut Cream (page 226).

mint: Try steeping fresh mint in hot water for a refreshing fresh mint tea (also great for soothing an upset stomach).

thyme: I love me some thyme in any mushroom dish. Bonus: Thyme oil is an antimicrobial, which means it helps fight germs and is thought to soothe a sore throat.

dill: The smell of fresh dill always means good things are cooking. One of my favorite ways to incorporate the pungent herb is in Green Goddess Dressing (page 168).

FRUIT

berries: So good for you (all of those antioxidants) and so delicious. I try to keep on hand fresh or frozen blueberries, raspberries, blackberries, and strawberries for smoothies and snacking.

pineapple: Great in a smoothie, a cocktail, in chia pudding, or all on its own. Try to buy fresh or frozen, as canned pineapple can get soggy.

pears: When in season, I love a sliced pear with a nice nut cheese and some crackers.

apples: My year-round go-to snack with almond butter.

mangoes: Straight up, in salad, or as part of my Braised Chipotle Chicken (page 190).

melons: Hydrating and low in sugar, melons are a pain in the butt to butcher, but you will always be glad to see those refreshing cubes in your fridge.

papaya: I love the flavor of papaya, and it contains an enzyme that aids digestion. Add it to smoothies for flavor and a massive hit of vitamin C. Just be sure to buy organic—there is a lot of GMO papaya out there.

OILS AND CONDIMENTS

sesame oil: If you love Asian food as much as I do, and you want to make my Thai Lemongrass Soup (page 136), pick up some sesame oil if you don't have it already.

coconut oil: I use coconut oil liberally as a moisturizer as well as an ingredient in cooking—and in my morning lattes!

olive oil: This is my go-to oil—rich, grassy, good for cooking and drizzling in equal measures.

MCT oil: Great in coffee, tea, and smoothies. MCT stands for medium-chain triglycerides. This kind of saturated fatty acid is a brain booster and fat burner, and it is a key ingredient in my morning latte ritual (page 54).

ghee: I sub this clarified butter for regular butter basically always, but especially when cooking with high heat.

avocado oil: This mildly flavored oil is a great cooking oil, and it's high in vitamin E, which makes it excellent for skin.

apple cider vinegar: Stir it into your Bone Broth Base (page 127) and Dijon Don dressing (page 167).

balsamic vinegar: Great for a quick dressing with olive oil and essential with fresh tomatoes and basil or if you want to make a balsamic reduction (page 115).

fish sauce and/or ponzu: The perfect punch of acidity to liven up Asian-Style Dressing (page 166).

Sriracha: yes, please.

miso: Seasons my Walnut-Lentil Pâté (page 140) and makes the easiest "insta-soup" in town (stir a spoonful into hot water, and add some tofu and scallions for good measure).

coconut aminos: Just another thing coconut rocks at: being soy sauce. Coconut aminos are like soy sauce without the possibility that you'll consume any GMOs. Made from coconut sap and sea salt, this is a liquid that is rich with umami kick, has no gluten, and is MSG-free.

MY FAVORITE FEEL-GOOD SWAPS

I love chocolate, I love pasta sauces, I love milks. But I don't love dairy and I don't love gluten. So I make a swap. Milk chocolate, no thanks. Dark chocolate, yes, please.

I like a sweet. I like a snack. I'm not going to apologize for that! I'm going to figure out a way to make it work! What I know is that you can be healthy and still get your sweet or savory cravings fully fulfilled, because whatever you love, there's bound to be a healthier version out there

that satisfies the same urges. And I'm not talking about a disappointing chemical substitute. I'm talking about a swap that really satisfies.

For instance, I love the experience of a huge bowl of pasta with sauce. And I can still have my Bolognese and feel good, too (page 200). I can still have dessert. I can still have a sandwich. I can still have a sweet, creamy latte.

And so can you.

INSTEAD OF	FEEL GOOD WITH
Candy bars that contain corn syrup, sugar, artificial flavors, and colors.	Dark chocolate, which contains antioxidant groups like flavonoids, which are good for your heart, and polyphenols, which are good for your cholesterol levels.[6]

INSTEAD OF	FEEL GOOD WITH
Dairy milk, which is not always great for the digestive system of adult humans (especially this adult human).	Nut milks, which take on the nutritional profile of whatever nut you're using. Almonds can lower blood sugar levels,[7] cashews have magnesium, which is important for bones and muscles,[8] macadamia nuts protect against inflammation. And all these nuts have protein and are packed with vitamins and minerals.

INSTEAD OF	FEEL GOOD WITH
White flour pasta, which is made from refined white flour	Zoodles including carrot, zucchini, or sweet potato; bean, lentil, or chickpea pasta; or kelp noodles.

INSTEAD OF	FEEL GOOD WITH
Fat-free dairy yogurt, which researchers have discovered is missing something crucial for your health—fat!!	Coconut yogurt: delicious and full of healthy fat and probiotics, as well as protein, calcium, and B_{12}. Whole-milk yogurt: See page 94 for why it's the way to go if you're eating dairy yogurt.

INSTEAD OF	FEEL GOOD WITH
White bread, which is just more refined flour, still stripped of nutrition during processing, still not good for you.	Sprouted-seed bread: sprouting makes the minerals and vitamins extra available for your body so you can make your sandwich dreams come true and still get maximum nutrition on the side.

INSTEAD OF	FEEL GOOD WITH
Artificial sweeteners or processed sugar.	Coconut palm sugar or monk fruit sweetener.
Fruit juice, which strips out all of the fiber, since fiber is what keeps the natural sugars in fruit from torpedoing your system.	Fruit, which offers a host of vitamins, minerals, antioxidants, and a natural balance of fiber and sugars that gives you energy without the sugar overload.
Soda—which is full of corn syrups and other mysterious ingredients you can't pronounce. And really, all that sugar just turns into fat in your liver (gross) and contributes to belly fat.[9]	Sparkling water hit with a squeeze of lemon or lime, which gives you everything you need, and nothing you don't.
Parmesan—if you're ditching dairy completely, this has to go, too.	Nutritional yeast, which those in the know call "nooch." It's salty and delicious and also antiviral and antibacterial. Made of sugarcane and beet molasses and grown from tiny fungi, it's got no dairy, no gluten, just lots of protein and B vitamins. And it tastes nutty, cheesy, and kind of wonderful.[10]

THE WHOLE STORY ON WHOLE YOGURT

Yogurt is full of healthy probiotic bacteria that are crucial for a happy digestive system. Everyone agrees on that front. But there's been some confusion over the past few decades about low-fat vs. full-fat dairy products.

Here's the deal: The same era that gave us some truly great and lasting things—like David Bowie—also gave us some bad advice that we've still not quite dodged. In the '70s, we were told that low-fat (which is 4% to 5% fat) was better than full-fat, leading to nationwide consumption of watery coffee and runny, sweetened yogurt. By the '80s, the movement was in full swing, which was too bad because as we now recognize, those claims were not scientifically accurate.

To make it worse, manufacturers compensated for the diminished flavors in everything from dairy products to cookies by adding more and more sugar. Unfortunately, sugar accomplishes what fat was reported to do: It makes us fat. So hear this: Fat doesn't make you fat!! Too much processed sugar is what makes you gain weight!

Today, we still love David Bowie, but we can love our full-fat yogurt, too. Eating whole dairy products can actually help prevent weight gain[11] and diabetes. Fat helps you feel full, and it slows the absorption of sugars in your bloodstream. So if you're going to eat dairy yogurt with your berries, choose the stuff that is full-fat, full-delicious, full-satisfaction.

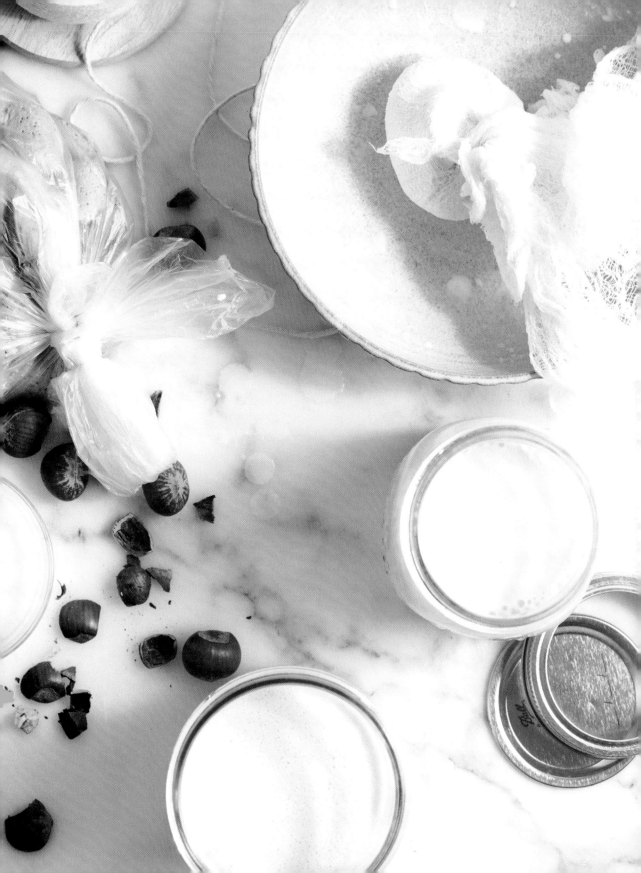

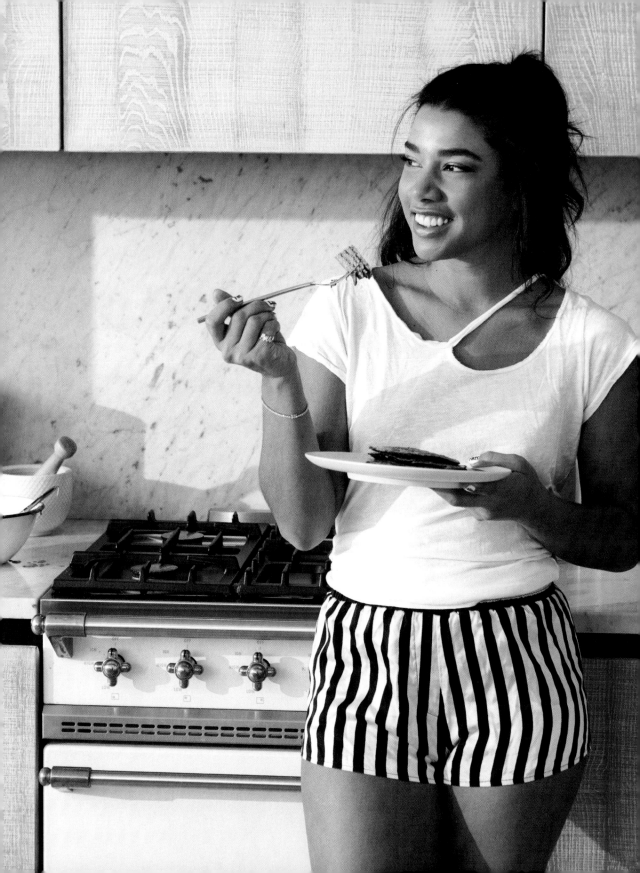

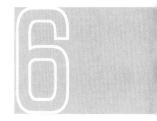

6

come and
GET IT

BREAKFAST FOOD FOR EVERY MOOD

CHIA PUDDING

Chia seeds are a bona fide superfood. They're high in omega-3 fats and packed with plenty of protein and fiber, making chia pudding a great way to start off your morning on the right foot. And it's incredibly simple to make: just follow the basic ratio of chia seed to milk, and add your favorite fruits and flavorings.

BASIC CHIA PUDDING

I love to make a batch of chia pudding on a Sunday and have it on hand for quick breakfasts and snacks during the week. I make mine with coconut milk, which is so sweet I don't need to add any sweetener, but you can use any nondairy milk you prefer. Be sure to give your jar a good shake before putting it in the fridge so the seeds don't get clumped together at the bottom!

Serves 1

1. Combine all the ingredients in a mason jar (or other glass container with a lid) and refrigerate for at least 6 hours; overnight is best.

2. Eat as is or check out the following variations.

INGREDIENTS

$\frac{1}{4}$ cup chia seeds

1 cup milk of your choice (almond, coconut, and pistachio are great choices)

1 packet stevia (or 5 to 6 drops liquid stevia)

$\frac{1}{4}$ teaspoon pure vanilla extract

THE ALMOND JOY

What happens when you combine creamy chia pudding with cocoa powder, coconut, and almonds? You get pretty close to the exact flavor of one of my favorite childhood candy bars. This chia pudding tastes like dessert but is low in sugar and high in protein, making it the perfect way to satisfy my sweet tooth without causing an insulin spike.

Serves 1

1. Once you've made the basic chia pudding, add the cocoa powder. Refrigerate for 6 hours; overnight is best.

2. Taste, and add stevia as needed.

3. Top with the coconut and almonds and enjoy!

INGREDIENTS

1 recipe Basic Chia Pudding (above)

1 tablespoon unsweetened cocoa powder

Extra stevia as needed

1 tablespoon unsweetened shredded coconut

1 tablespoon toasted slivered almonds

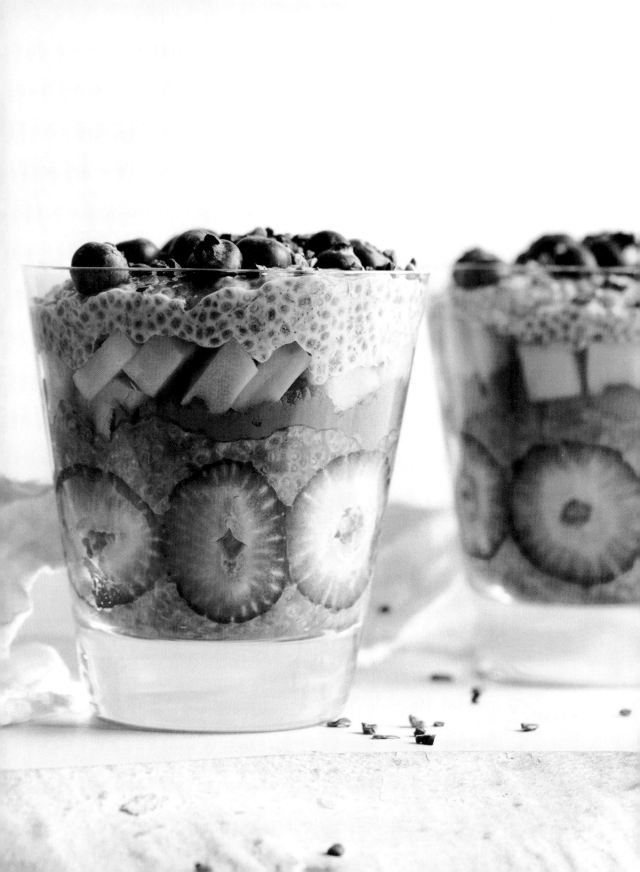

THE PARFAIT

This parfait requires a little assembly, but the final product is "Insta-worthy" and over-the-top delicious. Feel free to swap in whatever fruits you'd like—the more colorful, the better.

Serves 1

1. Make the basic pudding recipe and divide it in half between two bowls.

2. Mix the cocoa powder into one half of the Chia Pudding and let rest for 6 hours or overnight.

3. Mix the cinnamon into the other half and let rest for 6 hours or overnight.

4. When ready to serve, mix together the almond extract, the fruit, and the cocoa nibs.

5. In a glass or bowl, layer the chocolate pudding with half the fruit mixture. Top with the cinnamon pudding and the remaining fruit mixture and enjoy!

INGREDIENTS

1 recipe Basic Chia Pudding (page 99)

$1\frac{1}{2}$ teaspoons unsweetened cocoa powder

$\frac{1}{2}$ teaspoon ground cinnamon

$\frac{1}{4}$ teaspoon almond extract

$\frac{1}{4}$ cup diced strawberries

$\frac{1}{4}$ cup diced mango (or pineapple)

$\frac{1}{4}$ cup blueberries

1 tablespoon cocoa nibs

COCONUT YOGURT

Coconut yogurt is one of my favorite ways of getting probiotics into my body. It's fun to make and it's a great pre- and post-workout food. Coconut yogurt can be made in a few different ways. I've included two different ways to make it here: one uses frozen coconut meat, the other canned coconut milk. I make a big batch of this yogurt, which lasts for about two weeks in the fridge. I like to top it with fruit in the morning, mix it into smoothies, and even use it to make healthy desserts. In fact, it rarely lasts in my fridge for longer than a few days!

VERSION 1: FROZEN COCONUT MEAT

This yogurt is made using frozen coconut meat that you blend yourself to essentially make DIY coconut milk. I swear it tastes fresher and richer than canned coconut milk, the resulting yogurt has a nice tang and bite to it. It's delicious paired with fruit, nuts, or almond butter!

Makes 1¾–2 cups

1. Sanitize jars and lids using boiling water or your dishwasher.

2. Add the coconut meat, water, and lemon juice to a blender. Begin blending on low, gradually increase the speed to high, and blend until smooth.

3. Transfer to a small pot and heat over low to about 100°F. Monitor the temperature with a candy thermometer or digital thermometer if possible. If you don't have access to one of those, make sure the temperature is around the same temperature as your skin.

4. Make sure the milk is no warmer than 100°F (let cool if needed), then add the probiotics, salt, and syrup.

5. Mix to combine well, then transfer to the sanitized jars, and keep warm in an oven with the light on (to keep oven warm) or in a yogurt maker at 100° to 110°F. Leave for 12 to 24 hours.

6. Remove from the heat and refrigerate for at least 6 hours. At this point, the yogurt may separate—stir to recombine.

7. Keep refrigerated and use within 2 weeks.

Note: If a pink or gray film settles on your yogurt, it has become contaminated. Do not eat it.

*When looking for probiotic capsules, select something with the highest CFU count possible—either refrigerated or freeze-dried capsules are fine. Look for capsules that contain *L. bulgaricus, S. thermophilus,* and *L. casei* for best results.

INGREDIENTS

2 cups frozen coconut meat, thawed

½ cup coconut water or water

1 tablespoon fresh lemon juice

½ teaspoon probiotic powder (from probiotic capsules)*

Pinch of Himalayan sea salt

1 tablespoon pure maple syrup

VERSION 2: CANNED COCONUT MILK

INGREDIENTS

3 (14-ounce) cans full-fat coconut milk

$\frac{1}{2}$ teaspoon probiotic powder (from probiotic capsules)*

Pinch of Himalayan sea salt

1 tablespoon pure maple syrup

Coconut yogurt made with coconut milk is smooth, thick, and very rich. If you like a decadent yogurt, then this version is for you. It's full of high-quality fat, which is good for your brain, so you shouldn't be afraid of it. Remember, as with all things that are fermented, you need to give this one some time.

Makes 5–6 cups

1. Sanitize jars and lids using boiling water or your dishwasher.

2. Carefully scrape the thick cream off the coconut milk and transfer to a pot, along with about one-third of the milk.

3. Heat over low heat to about 120°F, stirring so the mixture combines well.

4. Allow to cool to less than 100°F, then add the probiotics, salt, and syrup.

5. Mix to combine well, then transfer to the sanitized jars, and keep warm in an oven with the light on (to keep oven warm) or in a yogurt maker at 100° to 110°F. Leave for 12 to 24 hours.

6. Remove from the heat and refrigerate for at least 6 hours. At this point, the yogurt may separate—stir to recombine.

7. Keep refrigerated and use within 2 weeks.

*When looking for probiotic capsules, select something with the highest CFU count possible—either refrigerated or freeze-dried capsules are fine. Look for capsules that contain *L. bulgaricus*, *S. thermophilus*, and *L. casei* for best results.

do
what
feels
good

PANCAKES

Who doesn't love pancakes? I basically grew up eating in diners (hey, I'm an NYC kid), and at any time of the day a stack of fresh, fluffy pancakes was always sailing by in some waitress's hand. Pancakes were an indulgence, but they were always worth it!

Since I don't like to deprive myself of foods I love, I found a way to make my fave morning meal a little healthier. Each of these pancake versions comes with a hefty dose of protein and is gluten- and refined-sugar-free.

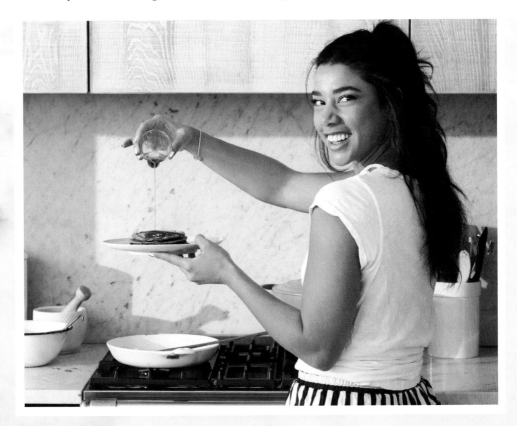

GREEK YOGURT PANCAKES

INGREDIENTS

1 cup oat, sorghum, or rice flour*

1 tablespoon baking powder

$\frac{1}{4}$ teaspoon ground allspice

$\frac{1}{4}$ teaspoon ground cloves

2 large eggs

$1\frac{1}{2}$ cups whole-milk Greek yogurt

6 to 8 drops liquid stevia

1 teaspoon pure vanilla extract

Grass-fed butter or coconut oil, for cooking

Greek yogurt makes these pancakes soft and tender. When I feel like eating dairy, this is one of my staples, but if you are avoiding it, you could swap in coconut yogurt or another non-dairy yogurt.

Serves 3 to 4

1. In a large bowl, whisk together the oat flour, baking powder, allspice, and cloves. Set aside.

2. In a separate bowl, stir together the eggs, Greek yogurt, stevia, and vanilla.

3. Fold the yogurt mixture into the dry ingredient mixture until well combined.

4. Heat a skillet over medium-high heat. Add the butter and reduce the heat to medium-low.

5. Spread about ¼ cup of the batter onto the skillet using the back of a spoon, until you've got a ¼-inch-thick pancake.

6. Cook 3 to 4 minutes, then flip and cook an additional 2 minutes.

7. Serve the pancakes with fresh fruit, or a little maple syrup.

*To make your own oat flour, grind oats to a flour-like consistency in a food processor or blender.

do
what
feels
good

PROTEIN PANCAKES

These are my amped-up pancakes—full of plant-based protein plus fiber and omega-3 fats from the flaxseed, supercharged with MCT oil. They're the perfect reward after a tough workout.

Serves 4

1. In a mixing bowl, combine the milk and flaxseed. Let sit for 5 minutes.

2. Add the oil, stevia, and vanilla to the flaxseed mixture and set aside.

3. Whisk together the protein powder, brown rice flour, baking powder, salt, nutmeg, and orange zest in a large bowl.

4. Add the wet ingredients to the dry ingredients and stir until just combined.

5. Heat a well-seasoned, cast-iron griddle (or ceramic-coated griddle) over medium heat. When the skillet is hot enough that a drop of water splashed on it sizzles and bounces, add about a teaspoon of coconut oil.

6. Scoop ¼ cup of the batter per pancake onto the skillet, leaving room for the pancakes to spread.

7. Cook 2 to 3 minutes, or until bottoms are set, before carefully flipping them. Cook another 3 to 4 minutes on the opposite sides until set.

8. Serve 2 to 3 pancakes per person, topped with fresh fruit and shredded coconut.

*If your hemp protein powder is on the gritty side, I suggest grinding it to a fine powder in a clean spice grinder or food processor so that it incorporates better.

INGREDIENTS

1 cup milk of your choice (almond or pistachio are my favorites)

3 tablespoons ground flaxseed

1 tablespoon MCT oil or melted coconut oil

½ teaspoon liquid stevia

½ teaspoon pure vanilla extract

½ cup hemp protein powder*

½ cup sorghum or brown rice flour

½ teaspoon baking powder

¼ teaspoon salt

¼ teaspoon freshly grated nutmeg

Finely grated zest of 1 orange

Extra coconut oil, for cooking

Fresh fruit and shredded coconut, for serving

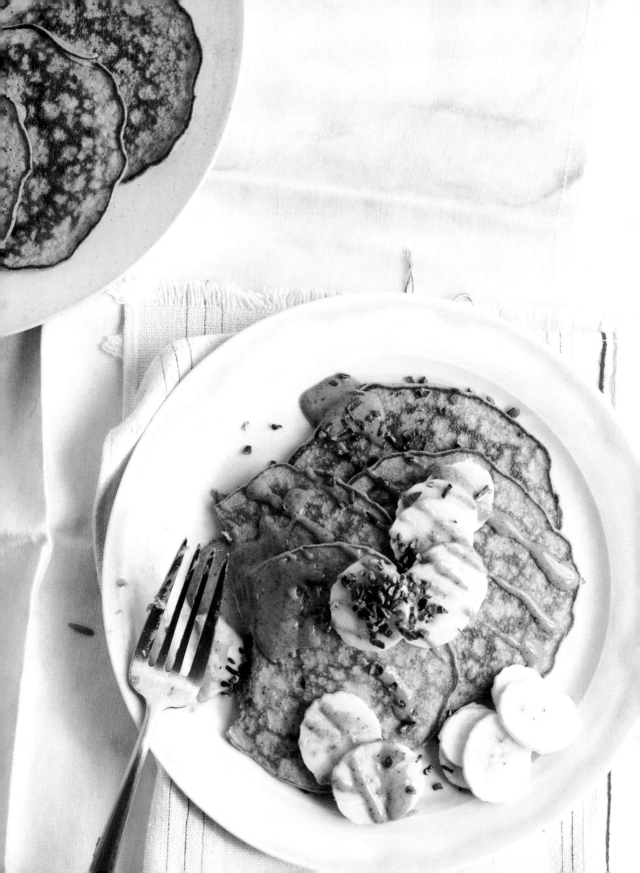

ALMOND BUTTER AND BANANA PANCAKES

Pancakes made of bananas and almond butter?? Enough said. The protein here comes from the eggs, which also give these sweet, nutty pancakes a light, crepe-like texture.

Serves 4

1. In a large bowl, mash the bananas until smooth.*

2. Whisk in the almond butter, then add eggs one at a time, making sure each is thoroughly incorporated into the mixture.

3. Stir in the cinnamon.

4. Heat a large cast-iron (or ceramic skillet) over medium-high heat. When the skillet is hot enough that a drop of water splashed on it sizzles and bounces, add the coconut oil.

5. Scoop 2 tablespoons of the batter per pancake onto the skillet, leaving room for them to spread.

6. Cook 2 to 3 minutes, or until the bottom is set, before flipping. Cook on the opposite side for an additional 2 to 3 minutes.

7. Serve topped with sliced bananas and cocoa nibs.

*I like to use a potato masher—if you want to make this even easier on yourself, you can make this recipe in a mixer or a high-speed blender—just add all the ingredients and process until combined.

INGREDIENTS

2 large, very ripe bananas

½ cup smooth almond butter

4 large eggs

1 teaspoon ground cinnamon

1 tablespoon coconut oil

Sliced banana and cocoa nibs, for serving

AVOCADO EGG CUPS

INGREDIENTS

2 large ripe avocados

4 large eggs

½ teaspoon salt

4 tablespoons chopped
fresh chives

Finely grated zest of 1 lemon

Hot sauce, for serving
(optional)

This super-simple dish combines two of my favorite foods: eggs and avocados. I often eat these egg cups for breakfast, but they also make for a quick and satisfying lunch. I love mine topped with a generous shot of hot sauce, but you do you!

Serves 4—or 2 very hungry people

1. Preheat the oven to 400°F.

2. Cut each avocado in half vertically and carefully remove the pits. If the pits are on the small side, you may need to carefully scoop out a little more space with a spoon—you'll want the hollows in the avocado to fit your eggs.

3. Arrange the avocados on a baking sheet, pit side up, using foil to keep them standing.

4. Crack the eggs into the hollows left by the avocado pits. Sprinkle with salt.

5. Carefully transfer to the preheated oven and bake for 15 to 20 minutes, until the egg whites are set.

6. Served topped with the chives, lemon zest, and hot sauce, if using.

do
what
feels
good

ZUCCHINI NESTS

Ever since I got a spiralizer I'm always looking for creative ways to eat more vegetables. I make zoodles a lot and eat them as pasta for dinner, but one day I thought, "I wonder how I could eat these for breakfast?" These cute little egg "nests" were the result!

Serves 4

1. Combine the zucchini and sea salt and spread out on a kitchen towel. Let rest for 15 minutes to draw out excess moisture.

2. Oil a baking sheet with the olive oil. Preheat the oven to 400°F.

3. Firmly pat the zucchini dry, then arrange in 4 tight "nests" on the prepared baking sheet, leaving a hollow in each for the eggs.

4. Crack 1 egg into the center of each zucchini cup, and top with the garlic, Parmesan cheese, and pepper.

5. Bake for 20 minutes, or until the egg whites are set and the zucchini is tender.

6. Serve topped with the fresh basil.

Want to make these for a brunch with friends? Try using oven-safe ramekins or even a large muffin tin for the nests. The final result is a perfect little nest. Your guests will be so impressed!

INGREDIENTS

4 cups spiralized zucchini (3 to 4 medium zucchini)

1 teaspoon sea salt

2 tablespoons extra-virgin olive oil

4 large eggs

2 garlic cloves, minced

4 tablespoons grated Parmesan cheese, or nutritional yeast

Cracked black pepper

Fresh basil, finely chopped, for serving

FRITTATAS

Frittatas are a great way to get a serving of veggies at your morning meal. They're also a great way to use up all of the lingering vegetables in your fridge. You can throw in whatever you have—anything goes once you have the basics down. I like to eat the leftovers for lunch or dinner with a nice green salad.

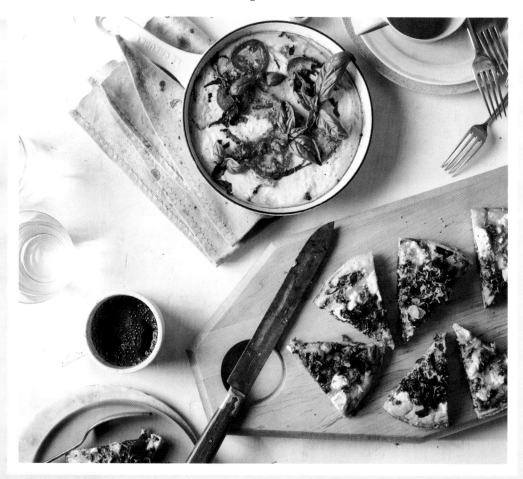

ALL THE GREENS FRITTATA

Multitask by putting your green salad in your morning breakfast instead of on the side. Feel free to swap in any green veggies you have on hand.

Serves 8

1. Preheat the oven to 350°F. Oil a 9-inch pie dish and set aside.

2. In a large bowl, whisk together the eggs and ¼ teaspoon of the salt. Set aside.

3. Heat a large sauté pan over medium heat. Add the olive oil, onion, and broccolini, and cook, stirring frequently, until tender.

4. Add the garlic, and cook an additional minute, until fragrant.

5. Add the kale, spinach, and parsley and cook until the greens have wilted. Remove from the heat and let cool to room temperature. Stir in the lemon zest and goat cheese, if using.

6. Add the greens mixture to the prepared pie dish, then top with the eggs.

7. Bake the frittata for 30 to 35 minutes, or until the eggs are set.

8. Serve topped with hot sauce, if desired.

INGREDIENTS

1 tablespoon extra-virgin olive oil, plus oil for the pie dish

8 large eggs

$1\frac{1}{2}$ teaspoons salt

1 onion, thinly sliced

1 cup finely chopped broccolini

4 garlic cloves, sliced

1 cup finely sliced kale

2 cups baby spinach

$\frac{1}{4}$ cup fresh flat-leaf parsley, chopped

Finely grated zest of 1 lemon

$\frac{1}{2}$ cup crumbled goat cheese (optional)

Hot sauce, for serving (optional)

HERBS AND 'SHROOMS FRITTATA

INGREDIENTS

1 tablespoon extra-virgin olive oil, plus oil for the pie dish

10 large eggs

$1\frac{1}{2}$ teaspoons salt

1 onion, finely diced

1 pound mushrooms (cremini, portobello, button, shiitake, or a mix), finely chopped

4 garlic cloves, minced

2 tablespoons fresh rosemary, finely minced, plus more for garnish

2 tablespoons fresh thyme, minced, plus more for garnish

Finely grated zest of 2 lemons

1 teaspoon freshly ground black pepper

$\frac{1}{4}$ cup shredded Parmesan cheese, or nutritional yeast (optional)

I love the earthy flavor of mushrooms, and I especially love mushrooms with a little bit of salt, thyme, and eggs—they just go so well together. I could eat a slice of this frittata any day of the week.

Serves 8

1. Preheat the oven to 350°F. Oil a 9-inch pie dish and set aside.

2. In a large bowl, whisk together the eggs and ¾ teaspoon of the salt. Set aside.

3. Heat a large sauté pan over medium-high heat. Add the olive oil, onion, remaining ¾ teaspoon salt, and mushrooms and cook, stirring occasionally, until the mushrooms have browned and onions are tender.

4. Add the garlic, rosemary, thyme, and lemon zest, and continue to cook an additional 2 to 3 minutes, until the mixture is very fragrant.

5. Remove from the heat stir in the pepper and Parmesan cheese, if using, then transfer to the prepared pie dish.

6. Pour the eggs over the mushroom mixture and bake the frittata for 30 to 35 minutes, until the eggs are set.

7. Serve garnished with the additional fresh herbs.

do
what
feels
good

MARGHERITA FRITTATA

Everyone loves a Margherita anything. So why not a frittata? If dairy's not your thing, you could use vegan cheese in place of the mozzarella. All you need is something melty and gooey to pair with the tomatoes and basil!

Serves 8

1. Preheat the oven to 350°F. Oil a 9-inch pie dish and set aside.

2. In a large bowl, whisk together the eggs and ¾ teaspoon of the salt. Set aside.

3. Heat a large pan over medium-high heat. Add the onions and the remaining ¾ teaspoon salt and cook, stirring occasionally, until the onions are tender.

4. Add the garlic and cook an additional minute, until fragrant, then add the tomatoes.

5. Cook over medium heat, stirring occasionally, until the liquid from the tomatoes has released and evaporated, then remove from the heat.

6. Transfer the tomato mixture to the prepared pie dish, along with the basil, mozzarella, and pepper. Stir to combine, then add the eggs.

7. Bake the frittata for 30 to 35 minutes, until the eggs are set. Serve drizzled with balsamic vinegar and garnish with the extra fresh basil.

*To make your own reduction, cook balsamic vinegar in a pan over medium heat until reduced and syrupy. Let cool before using.

INGREDIENTS

1 tablespoon extra-virgin olive oil, plus oil for the pie dish

10 large eggs

1½ teaspoons salt

2 onions, thinly sliced

4 garlic cloves, sliced

3 large ripe tomatoes, diced

1 cup finely sliced fresh basil, plus extra for garnish

1 cup shredded mozzarella cheese

1 tablespoon freshly ground black pepper

Balsamic reduction, for serving*

#HASH

Hash is such a comfort food for me that I was hell-bent on finding ways to make it more nutritious. I like to use a variety of root vegetables, including sweet potatoes, carrots, and beets in my hash. And topping it all off with an egg (or a few slices of bacon) for a nice dose of protein never hurts!

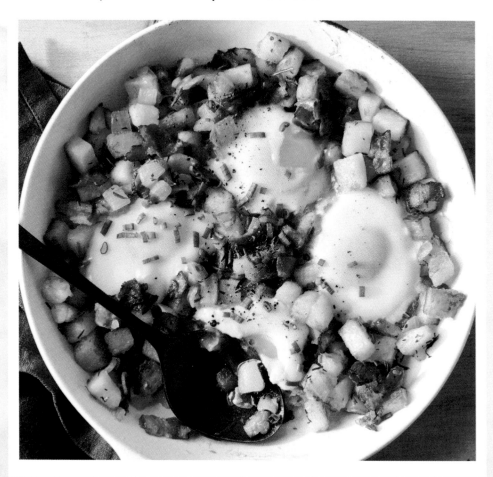

SWEET POTATO HASH

Bring on the root vegetables—these vibrantly colored ingredients make for a beautiful hash. And sweet potatoes are one of the most nutrient-dense foods around, while beets are prized for the boost they give to your brain and your heart. Hashtag win-win.

Makes 2 generous servings

1. Heat the olive oil over medium-high heat in a large sauté pan.

2. Add the onion, sweet potato, beet, and carrots and cook, stirring frequently, until the sweet potatoes and beets are super tender, 10 to 15 minutes.

3. Add the garlic, thyme, and orange zest, and continue to cook 2 to 3 minutes more, until the garlic is tender and fragrant.

4. Serve as is or use for Baked Eggs in Hash (page 119).

INGREDIENTS

2 tablespoons olive or avocado oil

1 diced red onion

2 cups diced sweet potato (about 1 large)

1 cup peeled, diced beet (about 1 large)

2 carrots, peeled and diced

2 garlic cloves, minced

1 teaspoon minced fresh thyme

Finely grated zest of 2 oranges

BACON, ONION, AND POTATO HASH

INGREDIENTS

4 strips nitrate-free bacon, thinly sliced

2 large onions, diced

2 medium russet potatoes, diced (2 to 3 cups total)*

1 tablespoon fresh rosemary, minced

1 teaspoon fresh thyme, minced

$\frac{1}{2}$ teaspoon sea salt

$\frac{1}{2}$ teaspoon freshly ground black pepper

$\frac{1}{2}$ cup sliced scallions

Bacon lovers: I feel you. Sometimes you just crave that salty-crispy-sweet satisfaction. This hash has it all—potatoes, onions, fresh herbs, and bacon. It's a decadent and delicious way to breakfast and brunch.

Serves 2

1. Heat a large sauté pan over medium heat. Add the bacon and cook, stirring occasionally, until the fat begins to render.

2. Add the onions and potatoes and continue to cook, stirring frequently, until the potatoes are tender, the onions are fragrant, and the bacon is crisp.

3. Season with the rosemary, thyme, salt, and pepper, and half the scallions and cook for 1 to 2 minutes more, until very fragrant.

4. Serve garnished with the remaining scallions or use for Baked Eggs in Hash (page 119).

*For a more refined presentation, feel free to peel the potatoes. Or leave unpeeled for a more rustic hash (with crispier edges).

do
what
feels
good

BAKED EGGS IN HASH

Want to make your hash a complete meal? Put an egg on it. You could just fry up an egg and throw it on top, but I love the texture of a baked egg, and the hash offers a perfect little base to soak up a runny yolk.

Serves 2

1. Preheat the oven to 400°F. Oil an 8-inch baking dish or pie dish with the olive oil.

2. Line the baking dish with the hash, making 4 hollows for the eggs.

3. Crack the eggs into the hollows and sprinkle with the sea salt.

4. Bake for 15 to 20 minutes, or until the egg whites are set.

5. Remove from the heat and serve sprinkled with the chives.

INGREDIENTS

2 teaspoons extra-virgin olive oil

2 cups hash of your choice

4 large eggs

$\frac{1}{2}$ teaspoon sea salt

$\frac{1}{4}$ cup sliced fresh chives or scallions

SMOKED FISH

My dad's side of the family is Jewish and I grew up eating lots of smoked fish. I remember being five years old and my mom entertaining—she would have me walk around with a little tray and serve tea sandwiches with smoked salmon to her guests. Smoked fish was usually in the fridge and always brought out for celebrations. To this day, anytime I eat it, I'm reminded of my family.

SMOKED TROUT MOUSSE

When I lived downtown, my best friend and I would go to the classic Jewish deli Russ and Daughters. We would get two sandwiches and split them both: an everything bagel with lox and scallion cream cheese, and a bialy with trout mousse. This mousse is my homage to those breakfasts!

Makes 4 ½-cup servings

1. In the work bowl of a food processor fitted with an "S" blade, combine the trout, cream, lemon zest and juice, horseradish, and black pepper.

2. Pulse until smooth, thinning out with additional cream, as needed.

3. When smooth, transfer to a bowl, and fold in the shallot.

4. Fold in the yogurt. Sprinkle with the reserved lemon zest and fresh parsley, if desired.

5. Serve as a dip for fresh veggies such as celery or bell peppers or spread mousse onto crackers or toast.

*If smoked trout is a little too "trout-y" for you, you can also try this recipe with smoked salmon—add a little minced dill to really enhance the flavor.

INGREDIENTS

8 ounces smoked trout*

¼ cup heavy cream or unsweetened coconut cream, plus 2 to 3 tablespoons, or as needed

Finely grated zest and juice of 1 lemon (reserve some zest for serving)

2 tablespoons grated horseradish (fresh or prepared)

1 tablespoon freshly ground black pepper

¼ cup very finely diced shallot or red onion

1 cup plain coconut yogurt, Greek yogurt, or room-temperature cream cheese (your choice!)

Handful of fresh parsley

AVOCADO-SMOKED SALMON TOAST

INGREDIENTS

1 ripe avocado

Finely grated zest and juice of 1 lemon

$\frac{1}{4}$ teaspoon ground cumin

$\frac{1}{2}$ teaspoon sea salt

4 slices rye or pumpernickel bread, toasted

2 tablespoons capers

1 tablespoon minced red onion

1 cup arugula

4 ounces sliced smoked salmon

This smoked salmon toast is a grown-up version of what I used to have back in the day. If you don't like rye or pumpernickel bread, you could use Ezekiel sprouted grain bread instead.

Serves 2

1. In a bowl, mash the avocado with the lemon zest and juice, cumin, and salt.

2. Spread the avocado mixture on the toast, and top with the capers, red onion, and arugula.*

3. Top with the smoked salmon, and serve.

*You can also put the capers, onion, and arugula on top of the salmon, but layering them between the salmon and the avocado makes this dish easier to eat!

do
what
feels
good

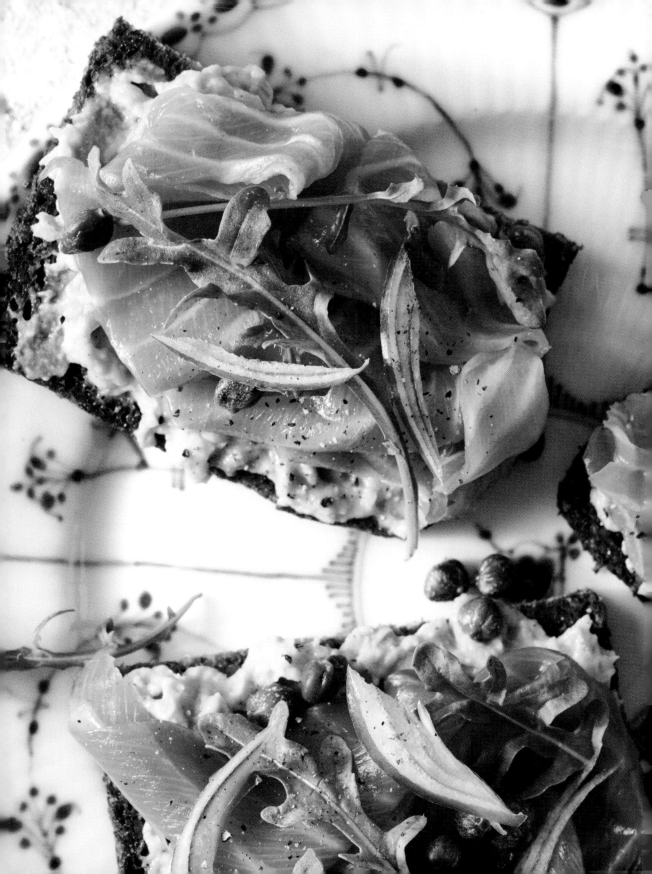

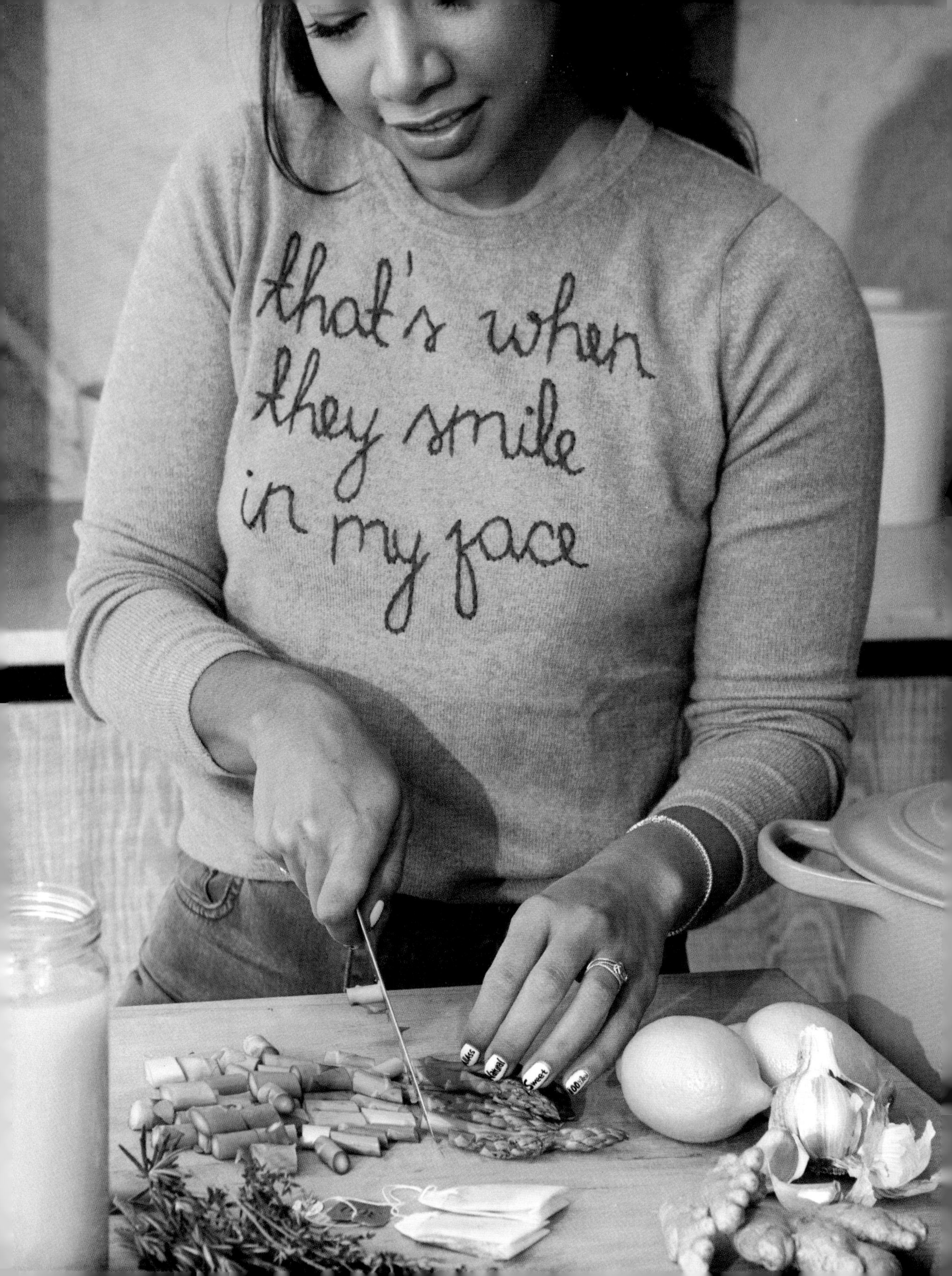
that's when
they smile
in my face
Sweet

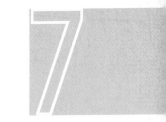

BROTH
FOR days

SOUPS AND OTHER LIQUID MAGIC

BROTHS

There's a lot of buzz about bone broth right now, so you might (rightly) wonder: What exactly *is* bone broth? Is it just the watery, salty base of your chicken soup? Why is it so "healthy"? Do you have to buy it at a fancy soup place or can you make it at home?

I've gotten into the bone broth craze myself, not because it's trendy but because it's delicious and the benefits are real. The collagen is supposed to be great for people who have or want to prevent leaky gut. (That is definitely me.) And bone broths offer a host of rich nutrients, including glucosamine, which protects joints (and as someone who loves fitness and uses my body hard, I am very into this). Bone broth also contains magnesium and calcium, which helps strengthen your bones, and it's great for your immune system overall.[1]

The recipe that follows can be tailored to your liking. Broth is only "bone broth" if it uses animal bones, but you can also make a delicious vegetarian or vegan broth using umami-rich mushrooms. It won't contain collagen, but it will contain plenty of vitamins and minerals.

BONE BROTH BASE

I like to sip this bone broth straight from a mug, like a cup of tea. I also use it as a base for other soups. It will keep in the freezer for up to 3 months, so don't be afraid of the large yield! I've even poured extra broth into ice cube trays and, once set, stored them in a container in my freezer so I can pop a cube into whatever I'm cooking as needed.

Makes approximately 2 quarts

1. Add all the ingredients to a pressure cooker, slow cooker, or stockpot.

2. Cover the ingredients with water.

3. Cook according to the instructions below.

PRESSURE COOKER: Let come to pressure, and cook for 90 minutes, according to the instructions from the manufacturer of your pressure cooker. Release the pressure and move on to step 4.

SLOW COOKER: Cook for 10 hours, covered, on low, then move on to step 4.

STOCKPOT: Cook, covered, for 6 to 8 hours over low heat, then move on to step 4.

4. Remove the bones and strain the broth through a strainer into a heatproof container. Strain a second time (through a fine-mesh sieve) to remove sediment, then use immediately, or refrigerate until using.*

*If you've used bones, this broth should gel in the refrigerator—that's a sign you extracted lots of collagen from the bones—don't be alarmed.

INGREDIENTS

4 pounds bones and gelatinous beef or chicken parts, such as chicken feet, neck bones, and thighs or beef marrow bones, short rib, and knuckle

5 celery stalks, roughly chopped

1 carrot, roughly chopped

1 medium white onion, unpeeled

5 garlic cloves, peeled

$\frac{1}{4}$ cup chopped fresh ginger, unpeeled

1 fennel bulb

5 sprigs thyme

1 sprig rosemary

Finely grated zest of 1 lemon

2 tablespoons apple cider vinegar or fresh lemon juice

2 to 3 bay leaves

1 tablespoon salt

Water; enough to cover the bones, no more than two-thirds of the capacity of your pressure cooker or three-quarters of the capacity of your slow cooker or stockpot

VEGGIE BROTH BASE

INGREDIENTS

2 pounds fresh mushrooms (any variety is okay)

5 celery stalks, roughly chopped

1 carrot, roughly chopped

1 medium white onion, unpeeled

5 garlic cloves, peeled

$\frac{1}{4}$ cup chopped fresh ginger, unpeeled

1 fennel bulb

5 sprigs fresh thyme

1 sprig fresh rosemary

Finely grated zest of 1 lemon

2 tablespoons apple cider vinegar or fresh lemon juice

2 to 3 bay leaves

1 tablespoon salt

Water; enough to cover the bones, no more than two-thirds the capacity of your pressure cooker or three-quarters of the capacity of your slow cooker or stockpot.

This broth is the perfect way to ward off the chill on a cold day. I like to heat up a bowl and add fresh greens and maybe some udon or soba noodles for a hearty, super-satisfying meal.

While a mushroom broth doesn't *need* all those hours of cooking, I find a long cooking time ideal for the meatiest flavor. I've given you some big windows for cooking times below! Customize your approach based on your patience and how soon you want to eat.

Makes about 2 quarts

1. Add all the ingredients to a pressure cooker, slow cooker, or stockpot.

2. Cover the ingredients with water.

3. Cook according to the instructions below.

PRESSURE COOKER: Let come to pressure, and cook for 30 minutes, according to the instructions from the manufacturer of your pressure cooker. Release the pressure, then move on to step 4.

SLOW COOKER: Cook for 4 hours, covered, on low, then move on to step 4.

STOCKPOT: Cook, covered, for 2 hours over low heat, then move on to step 4.

4. Strain the broth through a strainer into a heatproof container. Strain a second time (through a fine-mesh strainer) to remove sediment, then use immediately, or refrigerate until using.

A VERY GREEN GINSENG SOUP

This is an amped-up green soup for those looking to function in over-drive. Ginseng is great for your memory and clarity, and green tea gives you energy and helps keep your gut happy. Add some prebiotic asparagus, fresh herbs, and a hit of fresh citrus, and you've got a bowl of green goodness that will make you glow from the inside out.

Serves 4

1. In a large stockpot, heat the olive oil over medium-low heat.

2. Add the asparagus, ginger, garlic, and rosemary, and cook, stirring frequently, until the mixture is fragrant and the asparagus is tender.

3. Add the tea, basil, mint, thyme, lemon zest and juice, and stir until well combined.

4. Add the bone broth and let simmer for 10 to 15 minutes before serving.

INGREDIENTS

$\frac{1}{4}$ cup extra-virgin olive oil

2 cups chopped asparagus

$\frac{1}{4}$ cup minced fresh ginger or ginseng

4 garlic cloves, sliced

2 tablespoons minced fresh rosemary

Green tea from 2 tea bags

$\frac{1}{4}$ cup fresh basil

$\frac{1}{4}$ cup fresh mint

1 tablespoon fresh thyme

Finely grated zest and juice of 1 lemon

4 cups bone broth (page 127) or veggie broth (page 128)

THE SUPERGREEN

INGREDIENTS

$\frac{1}{4}$ cup extra-virgin olive oil

1 teaspoon sea salt

1 onion, diced

$\frac{1}{4}$ cup broccoli florets, chopped small

2 zucchini, diced

1 teaspoon dried basil

4 garlic cloves

$\frac{1}{4}$ cup fresh mint, chopped

2 tablespoons chopped fresh oregano

3 cups baby spinach

6 cups bone broth (page 127) or veggie broth (page 128)

1 cup frozen peas

Studies show that green vegetables can help protect you from skin cancer and breast cancer,[2] and we have stuffed this soup with the maximum amount of greens. This is a superprotective blend of veggies that delivers antioxidant overload, with plenty of A, C, and E, as well as folate, which is also important for cancer prevention.

Serves 4

1. Heat a large stockpot over medium-high heat.

2. Add the olive oil, salt, onion, broccoli, zucchini, basil, garlic, mint, and oregano. Cook, stirring frequently, until the zucchini is tender, the broccoli is bright green, and the onion is soft.

3. Add the spinach and bone broth and cook for 15 to 20 minutes, then add the frozen peas.

4. Cook for an additional 5 minutes and serve.

5. You can eat it chunky, but I like to blend it in my Vitamix! When blending in the Vitamix, I add a little bit of coconut cream.*

*Try whisking in a little coconut cream for a creamier soup or top it off with a little hot sauce if you like your food spicier.

do
what
feels
good

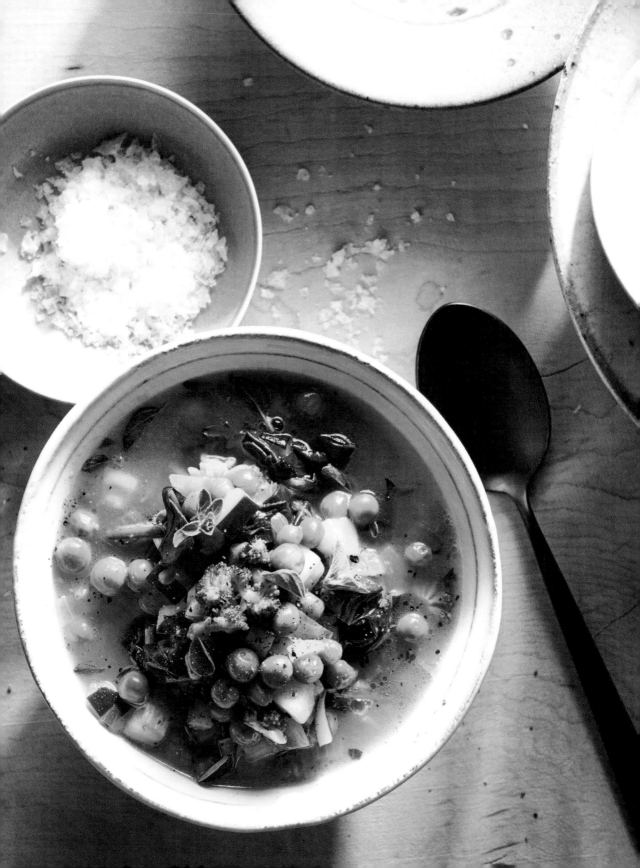

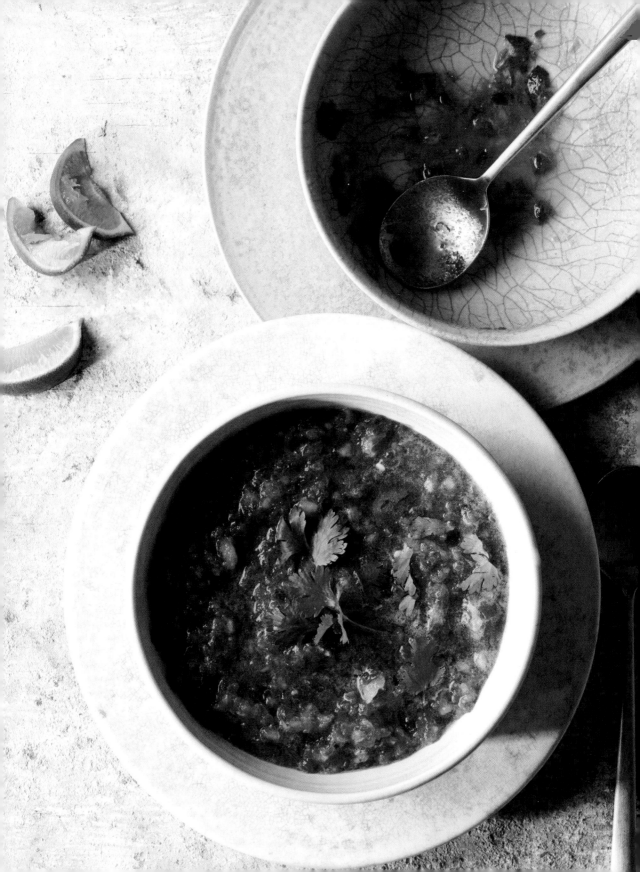

THE GAZPACHO

I've tasted many gazpachos in my day and I love them all. The best presentation I've experienced was in Italy, where they had all the veggies on a platter and you could add your choice into the chilled tomato base. It's so, so beautiful that way, but sometimes we don't have the time to make everything look perfect, in which case you just throw it all in the blender and call it a summer's day!

Serves 4

1. Add all the ingredients except the garnishes to a blender or food processor. and pulse until smooth.*

2. Taste, and add salt as needed

3. Serve cold, garnished as desired.

*You can also pulse until semismooth if you prefer a chunkier gazpacho.

INGREDIENTS

$\frac{1}{4}$ cup extra-virgin olive oil

$1\frac{1}{2}$ pounds ripe tomatoes

2 cups bone broth (page 139) or veggie broth (page 140)

1 cucumber, peeled

1 red bell pepper, stemmed and seeded

$\frac{1}{2}$ red onion

1 jalapeño

1 garlic clove

Sea salt

OPTIONAL GARNISHES

Tabasco sauce

Diced hard-boiled egg

Chopped jalapeño

1 cucumber, peeled and diced

Shredded cheddar cheese

Crumbled bacon

GREEN DETOX SOUP

INGREDIENTS

1 tablespoon avocado oil

1 large onion, diced

3 celery stalks, diced

2 cups kale, diced

½ cup sliced scallions

2 tablespoons minced fresh ginger

1 jalapeño, minced (seeded if you like it less spicy)

1 cup asparagus, finely chopped

4 cups bone broth (page 127) or water

Finely grated zest and juice of 2 limes

¼ cup fresh cilantro leaves

¼ cup fresh mint leaves

Sea salt

My green soup is the perfect meal if you just want to have a light meal that is nourishing and easy on your digestive system. It doesn't take a long time to make, and it packs a lot of nutrition into one bowl. I use bone broth as my base, but you can use veggie broth if you prefer. I like to top my bowl with a little coconut yogurt and extra lime zest for some creaminess and tang.

Serves 4

1. Heat the avocado oil in a large stockpot over medium-high heat.

2. Add the onion and celery and cook, stirring frequently, until tender.

3. Add the kale, scallions, ginger, jalapeño, and asparagus and cook until the kale has completely wilted and the whole mixture is very fragrant.

4. Add the bone broth and simmer for 15 to 20 minutes.

5. Transfer the mixture to a blender* along with the lime zest and juice, cilantro, and mint and blend until smooth.

6. Taste, and add salt as needed. Serve hot.

*If you prefer a chunky soup, you can skip the blending. Just mix in the lime zest and juice, cilantro, and mint before eating.

do
what
feels
good

COCONUT MILK SOUP BASE

When I traveled to Thailand a couple of years ago with my family, I found a lot of things that delighted me about the food there—first and foremost, how fresh and flavorful everything was. But I also loved how prevalent soup was, even though it was so hot, because I love soup. And I especially love it if it's made with coconut milk. Once you master this simple recipe, you can use it as a building block for any number of delicious soups.

Makes about 2 quarts

1. Heat the sesame oil in a large stockpot over medium-high heat.

2. Add the ginger, garlic, and shallots and cook, stirring frequently, until the shallots are tender, and the garlic and ginger are fragrant.

3. Add the coconut cream, coconut milk, and bone broth, and simmer for 15 to 20 minutes.

4. Remove from the heat, strain into a heatproof container, and whisk in the coconut aminos.

5. Store in the fridge for up to 1 week, or freeze for up to 3 months.

INGREDIENTS

$\frac{1}{4}$ cup sesame oil

$\frac{1}{2}$ cup sliced ginger (unpeeled is fine)

8 garlic cloves, chopped

4 shallots, minced

1 can coconut cream

2 (13.5-ounce) cans full-fat coconut milk

2 cups bone broth (chicken works best) (page 127)

Dash of coconut aminos, tamari, or soy sauce

THAI LEMONGRASS SOUP

INGREDIENTS

$\frac{1}{4}$ cup toasted sesame oil

lemongrass 1 stalk, sliced

3 scallions, sliced

3 garlic cloves, thinly sliced

2 cups fresh shiitake mushrooms, sliced*

2 cups shredded chicken (optional)

1 small Japanese eggplant, diced

1 ripe plum tomato, diced

1 cup Thai basil leaves

5 cups coconut milk soup base (page 135)

Dash of coconut aminos

Sriracha (optional)

Juice of 2 limes

I once took a cooking class in Chiang Mai, Thailand, and we made a soup that was very similar to this. It's hot, spicy, tangy, and deeply satisfying. Lemongrass has a flavor that cannot be duplicated—kind of like lemon, but then there's something a little more perfumed about it—it's just really aromatic and delicious.

Serves 4

1. In a large stockpot, heat the oil over medium heat.

2. Add the lemongrass, scallions, garlic, shiitakes, chicken (if using), and eggplant and sauté until the eggplant is tender and the lemongrass is very fragrant.

3. Add the tomato and basil leaves, and cook an additional 3 to 5 minutes, until the tomato releases juices.

4. Add the coconut milk soup base and coconut aminos and simmer for 20 to 25 minutes.

5. Taste, and add more aminos and Sriracha if desired. Add the lime juice just before serving.

do
what
feels
good

THE CURRIED COCONUT

This is the kind of seafood stew I would travel 8,509 miles for. When it's simmering on your stovetop, your whole house will smell AMAZING. I like my soup a little spicy, but you can add more or less red curry paste to achieve your preferred level of heat.

Serves 4

1. Heat the oil in a large stockpot over medium-high heat. Add the lemongrass, garlic, and the shallot and cook until the lemongrass and garlic are fragrant and the shallot is tender.

2. Add the curry paste and sauté for 1 minute. Stir to combine with the lemongrass, garlic, and shallot.

3. Add the coconut cream and cook until simmering, about 2 minutes.

4. Add the soup base and simmer for 15 minutes.

5. Add the shrimp and cook for another 20 minutes, then add the lime juice.

6. Serve garnished with the basil and cilantro.

INGREDIENTS

2 tablespoons sesame oil

2 lemongrass stalks, sliced

4 garlic cloves, sliced

1 shallot, thinly sliced

2 tablespoons Thai red curry paste

½ cup unsweetened coconut cream

5 cups coconut milk soup base (page 127)

1 pound shrimp, peeled and deveined

Juice of 1 lime

1 cup Thai basil leaves

½ cup fresh cilantro leaves

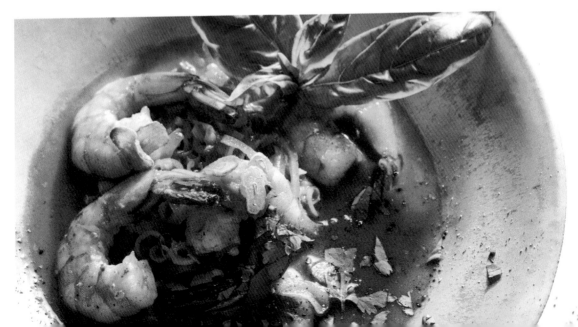

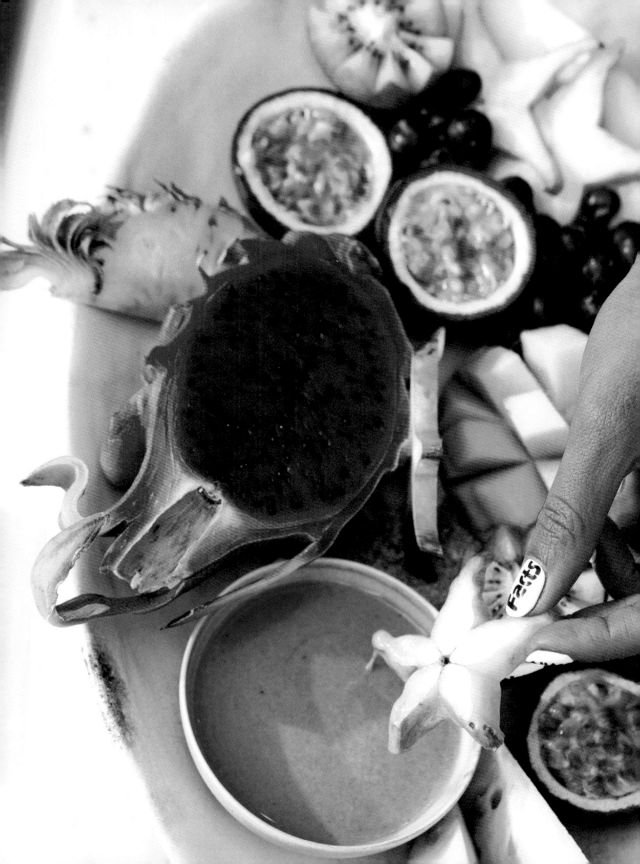

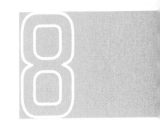

SPREAD ME on everything

BUTTERS AND PÂTÉS

WALNUT-LENTIL PÂTÉ

INGREDIENTS

1 tablespoon extra-virgin olive oil or walnut oil

1 large yellow onion, chopped

1 tablespoon fresh thyme leaves, minced

1 teaspoon minced fresh rosemary

1 tablespoon smoked paprika

1 teaspoon ground cumin

$\frac{1}{2}$ teaspoon salt, or more as needed

2 tablespoons white miso paste

1 tablespoon nutritional yeast

Juice of $\frac{1}{2}$ lemon

$\frac{3}{4}$ cup raw walnuts

1 cup cooked green or red lentils (or BPA-free canned lentils)

Nut spreads are simple to make and are a great alternative to cheesy or creamy dips. I like to serve them as part of an appetizer spread when I'm entertaining, and everyone always goes crazy for them.

Makes about 2 cups

1. In a large sauté pan, heat the olive oil over medium heat.

2. Add the onion, thyme, and rosemary and cook, stirring occasionally until the onion is tender.

3. Add the paprika, cumin, salt, and miso paste and cook an additional minute, until well combined.

4. Remove from the heat and transfer to a food processor fitted with an "S" blade.

5. Add the nutritional yeast, lemon juice, walnuts, and cooked lentils and blend until smooth.

6. If needed, drizzle in a little extra olive oil, until you achieve a smooth, spreadable texture.

7. Serve warm or at room temperature.

do
what
feels
good

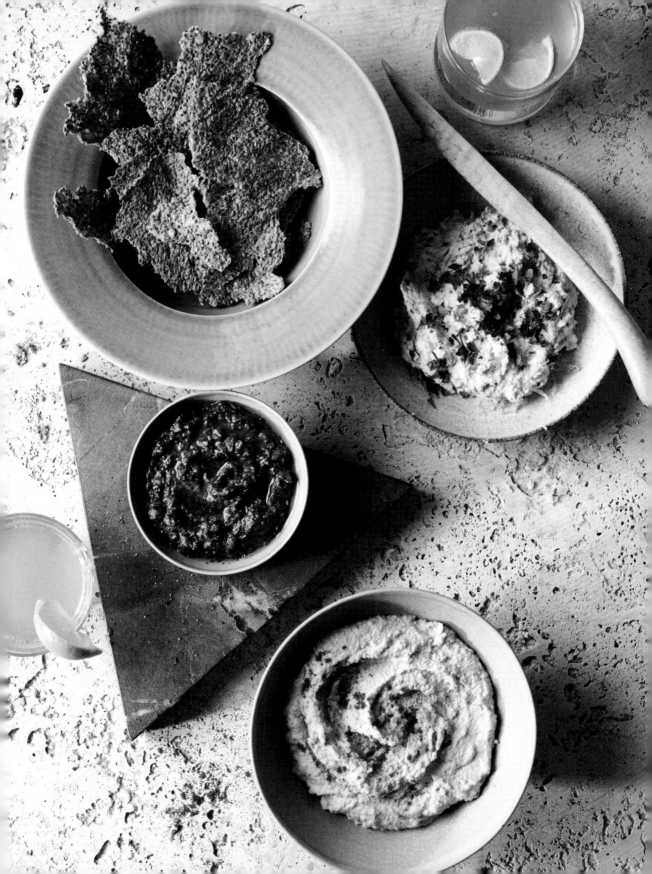

MORE-THAN-BASIC CRACKERS

INGREDIENTS

$\frac{1}{4}$ cup flaxseeds

$\frac{1}{4}$ cup chia seeds

$\frac{1}{4}$ cup sunflower seeds

$\frac{3}{4}$ cup water

OPTIONAL GARNISHES

Sea salt

Garlic powder

Minced fresh rosemary

Poppy seeds

Everything Bagel seasoning

What's a dip without a cracker? Sure, you can pick up a box of gluten-free crackers at just about any supermarket these days, but when I have the time, I love to make my own grain-free crackers. They're full of fiber, protein, and omega-3 fats, and they are super delicious!

Makes 3–4 servings

1. In a spice grinder, food processor, or high-speed blender, pulse the flaxseeds, chia seeds, and sunflower seeds until powdery.

2. Transfer to a bowl and add the water. Let sit for 20 to 30 minutes until congealed.

3. Preheat the oven to 300°F. Line a baking sheet with parchment paper.

4. Spread out the cracker batter in a thin layer on the parchment, and transfer to the oven.

5. Bake for 30 minutes, then add any desired garnishes to the top of the crackers.

6. Bake an additional 15 minutes, then let cool.

7. Break into bite-size pieces and serve immediately, or store in an airtight container for 1 to 2 days. Make sure they're completely cool before storing or they will get soggy.

do
what
feels
good

SWEET OR SMOKY CASHEW CHEESE

This cashew cheese really scratches that itch for a nice, spreadable cheese for snacking on crackers. It has the perfect texture and just the right amount of spice. You can go milder with a sweet paprika or add a flavor kick with smoked paprika—whatever your heart desires!

Makes about 4 cups

1. Place all the ingredients except the water in the work bowl of a food processor fitted with an "S" blade.

2. Pulse until a gritty paste has formed, then blend until smooth and spreadable, adding water as needed, a tiny bit at a time. This will take 1 to 2 minutes, and between ¼ cup and ½ cup of water, but go slowly with the water.

3. Taste, and add additional lemon and salt as needed.

4. Store in an airtight container in the refrigerator for up to 1 week.

INGREDIENTS

2 cups raw cashews, soaked 2 to 10 hours in water.

4 tablespoons nutritional yeast

Juice of ½ lemon

1 teaspoon paprika (sweet or smoked, depending on desired cheese flavor)

1 teaspoon garlic powder

1 teaspoon freshly ground black pepper

1 teaspoon salt

Water, as needed

SPINACH PESTO SPREAD, VEGAN OR CLASSIC

INGREDIENTS

$\frac{1}{2}$ cup toasted pine nuts*

2 garlic cloves

1 cup fresh basil leaves

2 cups fresh spinach leaves

$\frac{1}{4}$ cup shredded Parmesan cheese or nutritional yeast

Extra-virgin olive oil, as needed (about $\frac{1}{4}$ cup)

Sea salt

Juice of 1 lemon (optional)

This spread is so good—it's basically a thicker, dip-like version of pesto. You can keep it classic and use Parmesan cheese or swap out the cheese for nutritional yeast to make it vegan. Either way, you can't go wrong!

Makes 1½–2 cups

1. In a food processor fitted with an "S" blade, or a high-speed blender, pulse the pine nuts and garlic until gritty.

2. Add the basil, spinach, and Parmesan, and pulse until a very thick paste has formed.

3. Gradually drizzle in the olive oil, a little at a time, until the mixture is spreadable.

4. Taste, and season with the salt and lemon juice as desired.

5. Serve as a dip for crackers and veggies or as a spread.

*If pine nuts are unavailable or very expensive in your area, use toasted slivered almonds instead.

do
what
feels
good

MACADAMIA-GARLIC-CHIVE SPREAD

This recipe is inspired by a spread I had in Hawaii. It uses macadamia nuts, which have a distinctive richness and sweetness. That dip was so amazing I just kept dunking carrot after carrot after celery after radish—I couldn't stop. It was that good. So is this version.

Makes 2 cups

1. Place the soaked nuts, water, and lemon zest and juice in a high-speed blender or food processor.

2. Pulse until combined, then blend until very smooth.

3. Add the nutritional yeast and garlic and blend until smooth and well combined.

4. Transfer to a bowl and fold in the chives, parsley, and salt. Serve with veggies or crackers for dipping.

INGREDIENTS

2 cups macadamia nuts, soaked in water 2 to 4 hours

$\frac{1}{2}$ cup water

Finely grated zest and juice of 1 lemon

$\frac{1}{4}$ cup nutritional yeast

1 to 2 garlic cloves, peeled and chopped

$\frac{1}{4}$ cup finely chopped fresh chives

$\frac{1}{4}$ cup finely chopped flat-leaf parsley

Sea salt

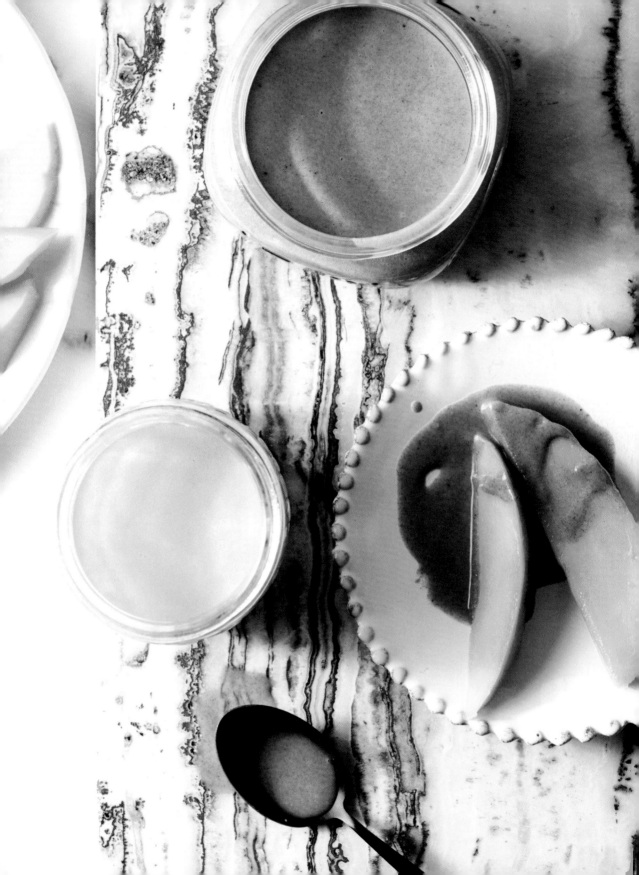

BLUE MAJIK BEAUTY BUTTER

I could eat coconut butter straight out of the jar (sometimes I do). But it's even better with the addition of superfood ingredients. Blue Majik is an extract of spirulina, which offers a beautiful hue and anti-oxidants for extra skin protection. Spirulina is a kind of blue-green algae that is one of the world's more incredible superfoods. It's great for detox and even helps fight candida. And pearl powder is amazing for the skin (that's why I call it a beauty butter). You'll get a hit of orange essence in each bite; choose honey or maple syrup if you like your butters on the sweeter side.

Makes 1 cup

1. Add all the ingredients except the coconut oil to the bowl of a mixer fitted with a paddle or a food processor fitted with an "S" blade.

2. Mix until well combined and creamy, adding the coconut oil, a teaspoon at a time, until you reach a spreadable consistency.

3. Serve with fruit or crackers or spread on toast. Store leftover butter in the fridge for up to 2 weeks; just let it come to room temperature and re-whip before using.

INGREDIENTS

1 cup coconut butter, at room temperature

1 teaspoon Blue Majik

1 teaspoon pearl powder (see page 62)

2 teaspoons raw honey or pure maple syrup (optional)

Finely grated zest of 1 orange

Coconut oil, as needed

PINK BEAUTY BUTTER

1 cup coconut butter, at
room temperature

1 tablespoon goji powder

2 teaspoons raw honey or
pure maple syrup (optional)

Finely grated zest of
1 orange

Coconut oil, as needed

With antioxidants for your skin and a reputation for making you feel calmer, this goji-powered butter is perfect for winding down after a big night out. Tart gojis can be eaten fresh or dried, and you can buy it in brightly colored (pink-orange) powder form at many health stores. To make it yourself, pulse dried goji berries in a food processor until you've made a fine powder. Add orange zest for a burst of citrus, and honey or maple syrup to adjust the natural tartness of the berries to your liking.

Makes 1 cup

1. Add all the ingredients except the coconut oil to the bowl of a mixer fitted with a paddle or a food processor fitted with an "S" blade.

2. Mix until well combined and creamy, adding the coconut oil, a teaspoon at a time, until you reach a spreadable consistency.

3. Serve with fruit or crackers or spread on toast. Store leftover butter in the fridge for up to 2 weeks; just let it come to room temperature and re-whip before using.

do
what
feels
good

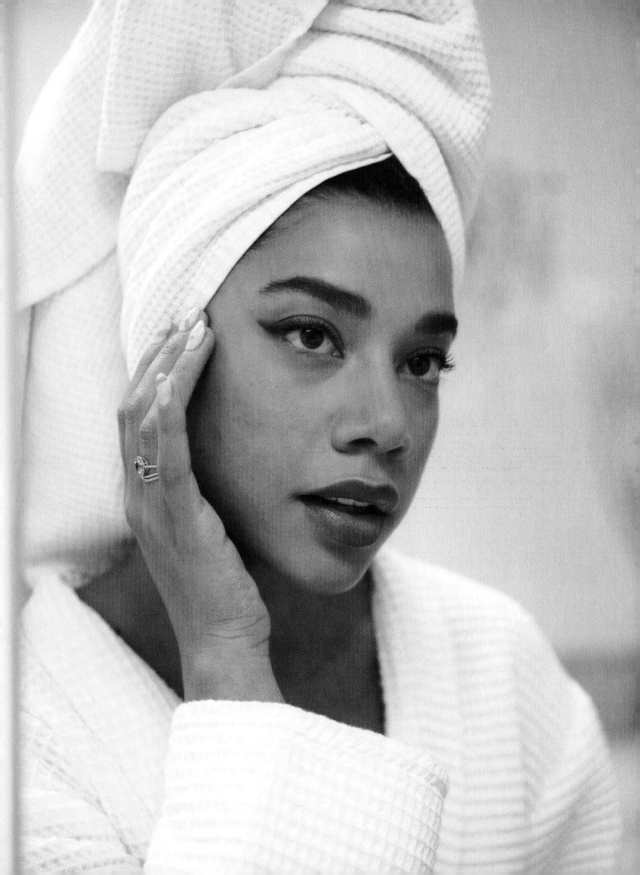

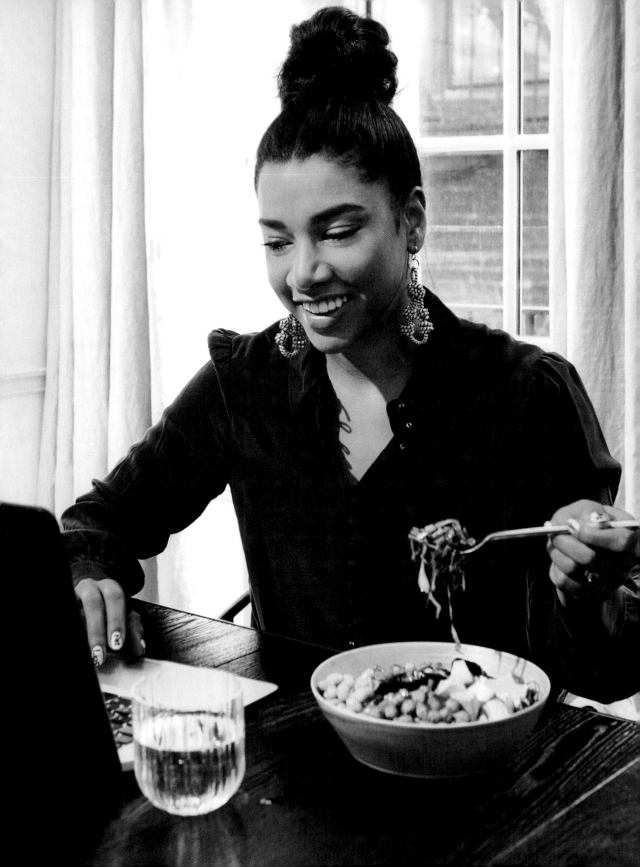

oneBOWL FITSALL

GET YOUR PROTEIN RIGHT HERE

GREEN BOWL WITH CHICKEN, CITRUS, AND HERBS

INGREDIENTS

$1\frac{1}{2}$ teaspoons extra-virgin olive oil

1 small shallot, minced

$\frac{1}{2}$ teaspoon sea salt

1 cup broccoli slaw

1 cup chopped asparagus

2 cups baby spinach

Finely grated zest of 1 orange

1 teaspoon za'atar

3 ounces leftover cooked chicken, shredded or finely chopped

$\frac{1}{4}$ avocado, pitted, peeled, and sliced

$\frac{1}{4}$ cup Green Goddess Dressing (page 168)

Finely grated zest of 1 lemon

$\frac{1}{4}$ cup minced fresh herbs (dill, parsley, mint, and tarragon work great!)

This warming bowl is packed full of veggies and protein, so it makes for an ideal midday meal to keep you satisfied. I'm absolutely obsessed with za'atar spice blend and put it on everything. In this case, when mixed with the citrus, it really gives this bowl a Mediterranean vibe.

Serves 1

1. Heat the olive oil in a large sauté pan over medium-high heat.

2. Add the shallot and sea salt, and cook, stirring frequently, until the shallot begins to turn translucent.

3. Add the broccoli slaw and asparagus and cook, stirring occasionally, until the asparagus is bright green and tender.

4. Add the spinach, orange zest, and za'atar and cook until the spinach has wilted. Add the chicken and cook until warmed through.

5. Transfer to a bowl, and serve topped with the avocado, dressing, lemon zest, and fresh herbs.

do
what
feels
good

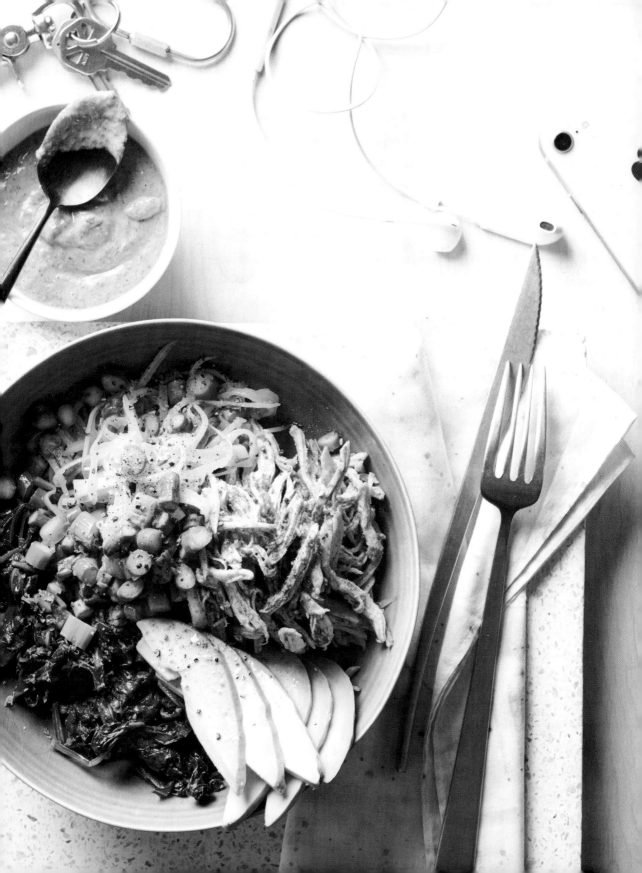

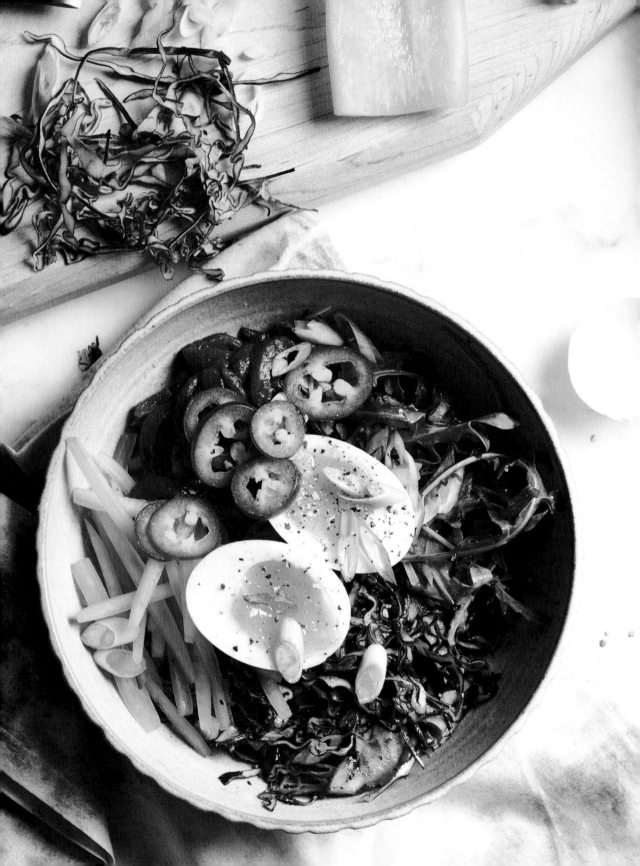

ANTI-AGING PEPPER BOWL

This crunchy bowl is packed with vitamin C, which is great for cell regeneration and helping protect our bodies from environmental damage. Yellow peppers also contain vitamin B$_6$, which is great for the skin.

Serves 1

1. Bring a pot of salted water to a boil.

2. Add the eggs and cook for 6 to 7 minutes for a soft yolk, or 10 to 12 minutes for a hard-cooked yolk. (A 6-minute egg is my favorite.)

3. Cool the eggs under cold running water and peel immediately. Set aside until needed.

4. Toss the cabbage, arugula, and mint with the Dijon Don and black pepper and transfer to a bowl.

5. Top with the yellow pepper, jalapeño, red pepper, and scallions.

6. Cut the eggs in half and add to the bowl just before serving.

INGREDIENTS

2 large eggs

1 cup shredded red cabbage

1 cup arugula

$\frac{1}{2}$ cup chopped fresh mint leaves

2 tablespoons Dijon Don (page 167)

1 teaspoon freshly ground black pepper

1 yellow bell pepper, stemmed, seeded, and thinly sliced

1 jalapeño pepper, thinly sliced (remove seeds to make it less spicy)

1 roasted red pepper, chopped

$\frac{1}{4}$ cup chopped scallions

SALMON BAHN MI BOWL

INGREDIENTS

1 tablespoon sesame oil

1 teaspoon peeled and minced fresh ginger

1 cup shredded kale

1½ teaspoons coconut aminos

1½ cups Cauliflower Rice (page 182), the cilantro lime variation

3 ounces poached salmon, flaked (see page 186)

½ cup shredded pickled veggies*

¼ avocado, pitted, peeled, and thinly sliced

1 tablespoon chopped fresh mint

1 tablespoon chopped fresh cilantro

1 tablespoon hoisin sauce

1 tablespoon hot sauce

A classic bahn mi sandwich is traditionally served on a baguette; this version takes the same flavor profile and packs in way more nutrients. Between the cauliflower, containing vitamin K, which is great for your blood, and the salmon, rich in omega-3 fatty acids, which are great for your skin and cells, this bowl is doing your whole body good.

Serves 1

1. Heat the oil in a large skillet over medium-high heat. Add the ginger and kale and cook, stirring occasionally.

2. When the kale has just wilted, remove from the heat, and splash on the coconut aminos.

3. Add the Cauliflower Rice to a bowl, and top with the prepared kale.

4. Top with the salmon, veggies, avocado, mint, and cilantro.

5. Drizzle with the hoisin sauce and hot sauce and serve.

*I like to pickle a mixture of shredded carrots, broccoli slaw, and thinly sliced red onions. To make them, heat ¼ cup of sea salt, 1 tablespoon pure maple syrup, and 2 cups of rice wine vinegar, whisking until the salt dissolves. Pour over the veggies in a heatproof bowl, let rest for 20 minutes, and serve.

do
what
feels
good

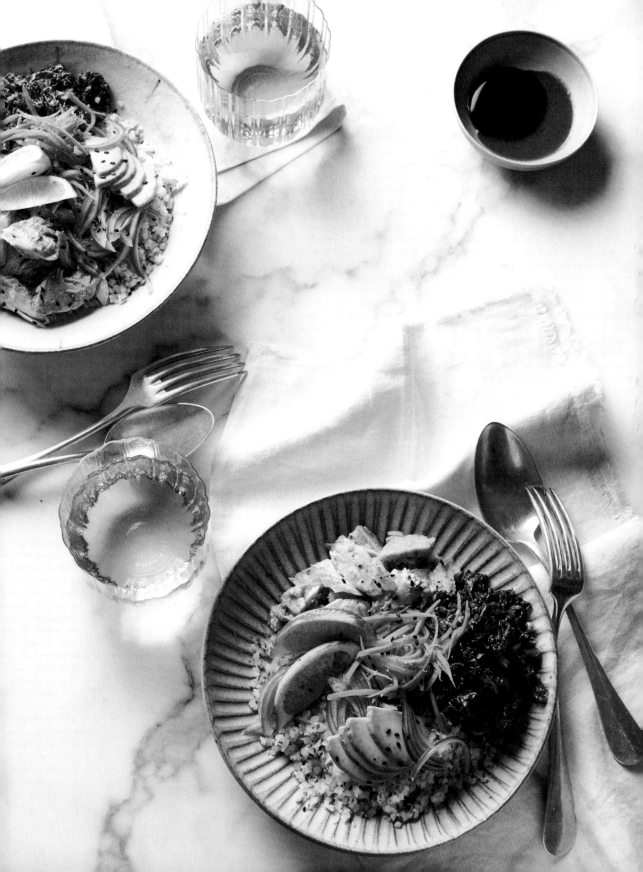

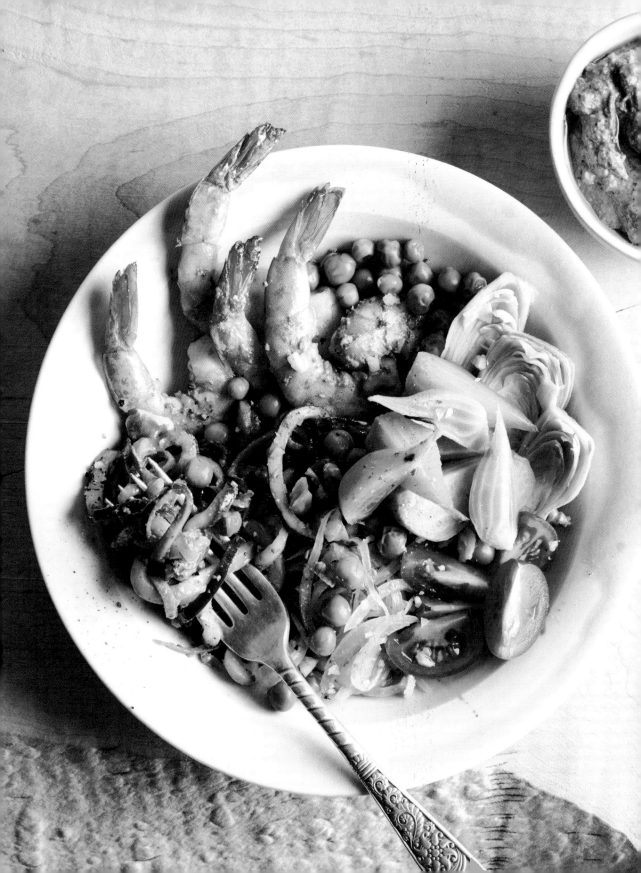

BODY BENEFIT BOWL

This tasty bowl does the whole body good. Artichokes contain gut-friendly prebiotic fiber, walnuts contribute brain-boosting omega-3 fats, and beets are packed with antioxidants that help you protect your cells from damage and fight inflammation. I like to add some garlicky shrimp to this bowl but feel free to omit if you prefer—you'll still get a nice hit of protein from the peas and walnuts!

Serves 1

1. Heat half the olive oil in a large sauté pan over medium-high heat. Add the noodles and cook with a pinch of salt for about 1 minute.

2. Add the onion and cook until the onion is tender. Toss with the pesto, and transfer to a bowl.

3. Heat the remaining oil over medium-high heat.

4. When hot, add the shrimp and garlic, and cook until the shrimp is just cooked through, 4 to 5 minutes.

5. Transfer to the bowl, along with the walnuts, tomatoes, artichoke hearts, beets, and peas.

6. Serve warm or at room temperature.

INGREDIENTS

1 tablespoon extra-virgin olive oil

2 cups zucchini noodles or carrot noodles (or a mix)

$\frac{1}{2}$ teaspoon salt

1 onion, thinly sliced

2 tablespoons pesto (see page 201)

3 ounces peeled and deveined shrimp

1 garlic clove, minced

2 tablespoons chopped walnuts

$\frac{1}{2}$ cup cherry tomatoes, halved

$\frac{1}{2}$ cup artichoke hearts, quartered

$\frac{1}{2}$ cup diced roasted beets

$\frac{1}{2}$ cup fresh steamed peas

SPICY VEGAN BOWL

INGREDIENTS

1 tablespoon avocado oil

$\frac{1}{2}$ cup cooked chickpeas
(canned and rinsed okay)

$\frac{1}{2}$ teaspoon sea salt

$\frac{1}{4}$ teaspoon chili powder

$\frac{1}{4}$ teaspoon garlic powder

2 cups shredded cabbage

2 tablespoons Asian-Style
Dressing (page 166)

1 teaspoon hot sauce,
such as Tabasco

$\frac{1}{4}$ cup cooked edamame
or peas

$\frac{1}{4}$ chopped avocado

$\frac{1}{4}$ cup chopped roasted beets

$\frac{1}{4}$ cup finely chopped
scallions

1 tablespoon roasted, salted
pumpkin seeds

This pretty bowl comes together easily and makes for a great vegan weeknight meal option. The edamame and chickpeas provide plenty of plant-based protein, and the dressing is to die for—I can put it on literally anything.

Serves 1

1. Heat the oil over medium-high heat. While the oil is heating, make sure the chickpeas are thoroughly dried.

2. Add the chickpeas, salt, chili powder, and garlic powder to the pan.

3. Cook, stirring frequently, until the chickpeas are golden brown and crispy.

4. Toss the cabbage together with the dressing and hot sauce and transfer to a serving bowl.

5. Top with the chickpeas, edamame, avocado, beets, scallions, and pumpkin seeds.

do
what
feels
good

SUMAC LAMB AND YOGURT BOWL

When Brendan and I went to Israel, the food was a huge part of our experience there. One of the best things we tried was the lamb kebabs—I ate them everywhere we went! After we came home, I couldn't stop thinking about and craving them, so I learned how to make them myself. For those of you who have never cooked with lamb before, this is a great starter recipe. Ground lamb is easy to work with—like any other ground meat—and the flavor of the herbs and spices complements the lamb perfectly.

Serves 1

1. Make the sauce by whisking together all the ingredients in a small bowl. Set aside.

2. Heat the oil in a small pan over medium heat. Add the lamb, sumac, sesame seeds, salt, and eggplant, and cook, stirring occasionally, until the eggplant is tender and the lamb has cooked through.

3. While the lamb is cooking, toss the tomato, onion, cucumber, and bell pepper together in a bowl.

4. Top with the eggplant and lamb mixture and a dollop of sauce and enjoy!

INGREDIENTS

FOR THE SAUCE

$\frac{1}{4}$ cup plain Greek yogurt (You can substitute dairy-free yogurt; just know it won't be as thick.)

Finely grated zest and juice of 1 lemon

1 tablespoon tahini

1 tablespoon minced fresh mint

1 tablespoon minced fresh dill

$\frac{1}{2}$ teaspoon sea salt

FOR THE BOWL

1 teaspoon olive oil

3 ounces lean ground lamb

$\frac{1}{2}$ teaspoon ground sumac

$\frac{1}{2}$ teaspoon sesame seeds

$\frac{1}{2}$ teaspoon sea salt

$\frac{1}{2}$ cup diced eggplant

1 large tomato, diced

$\frac{1}{4}$ sweet onion, minced

1 Persian cucumber, diced

1 yellow bell pepper, stemmed, seeded, and diced

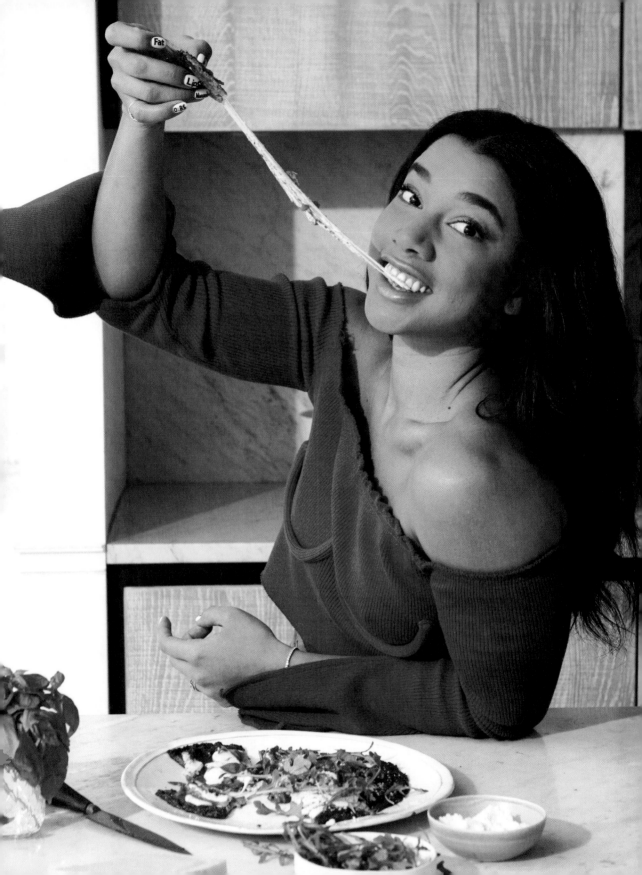

three
WAYS

ENTRÉES YOUR WAY

GREEN SALADS FOREVER

INGREDIENTS

2 cups of your favorite greens, torn into bite-size pieces

1 cup sliced raw fruits and/or vegetables of your choice (some of my favorites are carrots, cucumber, red onions, broccoli, cabbage, mango, apple, fennel, pomegranate, and blueberries)

$\frac{1}{2}$ cup fat or and/or protein (half an avocado, a hard-boiled egg, a handful of shredded cheese, a serving of fish or shrimp or chicken)

2 to 3 tablespoons salad dressing of your choice (see pages 166 to 168)

1 to 2 tablespoons crunchy toppings, such as sunflower seeds, crumbled crackers, almonds, or walnuts

Salads often get a bad rap, but I love a salad. I love the crunch of crisp greens, and I love that you can create so many different flavor profiles by pairing different ingredients and using different dressings. I try to always have my favorite greens on hand—usually spinach, arugula, baby kale—for a quick, simple salad. I throw them in a bowl with a handful of vegetables and then get creative with the dressing. This recipe isn't so much a capital "R" recipe as it is a ratio guideline for getting the balance of texture and taste just right. As with everything else in this book, it's all about customizing to create something that makes you feel good!

Serves 1

1. In a large bowl, combine the greens and fruits and/or veggies.

2. Add the dressing and toss to combine.

3. Serve topped with the toppings of your choice.

do
what
feels
good

DRESS IT UP

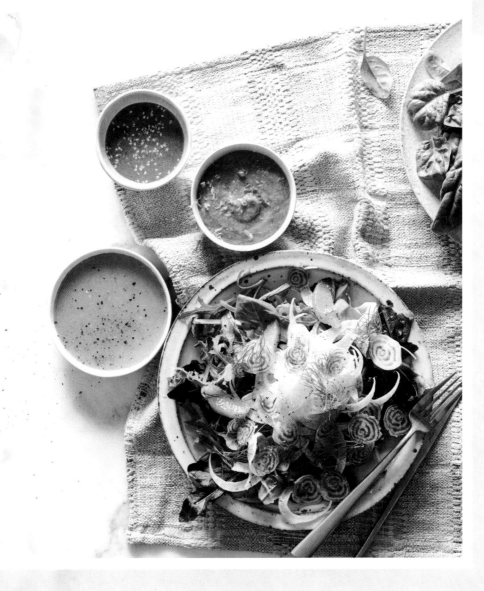

ASIAN-STYLE DRESSING

INGREDIENTS

2 tablespoons toasted
sesame oil

1 teaspoon fish sauce

2 tablespoons ponzu sauce

1 teaspoon coconut aminos

2 tablespoons almond
butter

1 tablespoon MCT oil

My favorite dressings tend to be those that include Asian ingredients like sesame oil and ponzu sauce and, of course, almond butter. This super-flavorful dressing is always on rotation in my house. You can use soy sauce in place of the coconut aminos, if you prefer, but if you're trying to avoid soy like I am, coconut aminos are a great alternative. This dressing is especially good with a spinach, mango, and cucumber salad combo!

Makes 4 servings

1. Place all the ingredients in a pint-size mason jar with a lid.

2. Shake vigorously until smooth.

3. Taste, and adjust the seasoning as needed—for more salt, add coconut aminos; for more acid, add ponzu; for a milder flavor, add MCT oil.

4. Store in the lidded jar in the refrigerator for up to 1 week. Let come to room temperature and give it a shake before serving.

do
what
feels
good

DIJON DON

This version of a classic Dijon dressing uses apple cider vinegar as its star ingredient, which offers a host of health benefits, including reduced blood sugar and cholesterol levels and even reduced belly fat. A nice hit of garlic offers immune support and a punch of flavor.

Makes 6 servings

1. In a small bowl, whisk together the vinegar, mustard, and garlic until well combined.

2. Drizzle in the olive oil gradually, until combined.

3. Taste, and add the salt and pepper as needed.

4. Store in a lidded glass jar in the refrigerator for up to 1 week. Let come to room temperature and give it a shake before serving.

INGREDIENTS

$\frac{1}{4}$ cup apple cider vinegar

$1\frac{1}{2}$ teaspoons Dijon mustard

1 garlic clove, crushed

$\frac{1}{2}$ cup extra-virgin olive oil

$\frac{1}{2}$ teaspoon salt, or more as needed

$\frac{1}{2}$ teaspoon freshly ground black pepper, or more as needed

GREEN GODDESS DRESSING

1 ripe avocado

1 garlic clove, crushed

Juice of 1 lemon

$\frac{1}{4}$ cup red wine or apple cider vinegar

2 tablespoons extra-virgin olive oil, plus more as needed

2 tablespoons minced fresh dill

2 tablespoons minced fresh parsley

2 tablespoons minced fresh chives

1 tablespoons minced fresh tarragon

1 teaspoon salt

I love a creamy salad dressing, and this rich, garlicky dressing made with avocado totally hits the spot. It pairs really nicely with a protein like chicken, salmon, or even a chopped-up hard-boiled egg. The fresh herbs make all the difference here (especially the dill!), but if you don't happen to have fresh tarragon on hand, you could use a teaspoon of dried.

Makes 8 servings

1. Place the avocado, garlic, lemon juice, and vinegar in a blender or food processor.

2. Blend on high until smooth, then drizzle in the olive oil until you achieve a smooth, pourable dressing consistency.

3. Add the fresh herbs and salt and combine with a few quick pulses.

4. Store in a lidded glass jar the refrigerator for up to 1 week. Let come to room temperature and give it a shake before serving.

do
what
feels
good

AVOCADO

When I visited my aunt in Australia, I ate the best avocados I've ever tasted in my life. It was on that trip that my love affair with avocados was truly cemented. Now they're a staple in my diet and my go-to source of healthy fats and fiber. Sometimes I find myself just eating an avocado on its own, scooping it right out of its skin with a little sprinkle of sea salt. When I decide to put in slightly more effort, these three recipes are my favorite ways of enjoying one of my favorite foods.

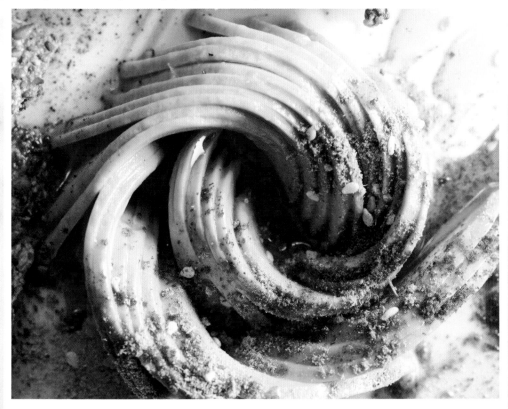

CALIFORNIA

INGREDIENTS

1 ripe avocado

$\frac{1}{2}$ teaspoon sea salt

1 teaspoon red chile flakes
(or more to taste)

Finely grated zest and juice
of 1 lime

More-Than-Basic Crackers
(see page 142)

If you're over #avocadotoast I feel you! This twist on the original offers great texture by swapping out bread (which, let's be real, often gets soggy under the weight of all that avocado) for More-Than-Basic Crackers (page 142). The result is an avocado cracker that can be shared as a snack or hoarded solo for a meal.

Serves 2

1. Cut the avocado in half lengthwise and remove the pit.

2. Remove the avocado flesh from the peel and place in a bowl.

3. Add the sea salt, chile flakes, and lime zest and juice and mix well to combine.

4. Serve on the crackers.

do
what
feels
good

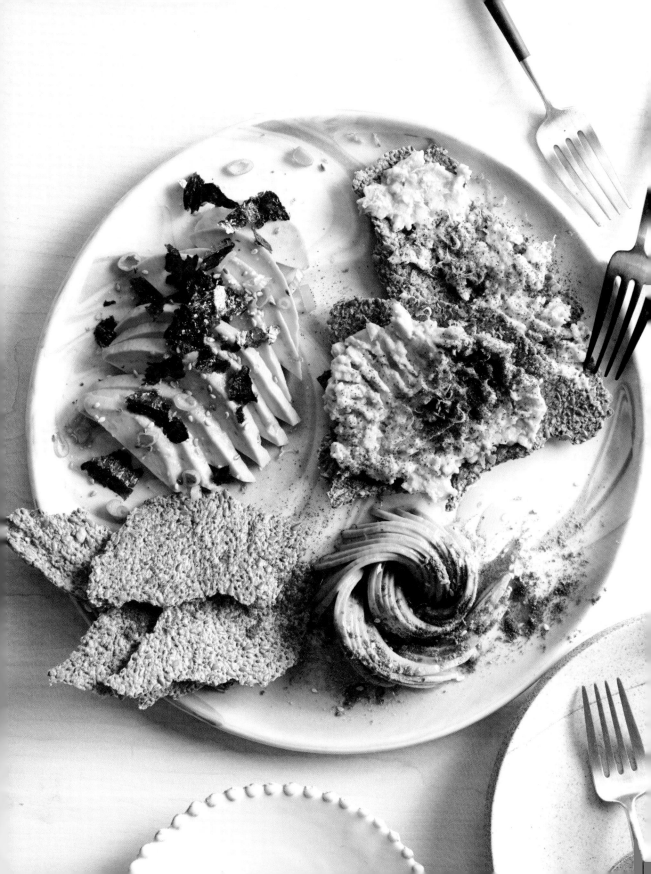

ZA'ATARVO (ZA'ATAR + AVOCADO)

INGREDIENTS

1 ripe avocado

2 teaspoons extra-virgin olive oil

2 tablespoons za'atar

2 teaspoons paprika

1 teaspoon sea salt

Finely grated zest of 1 lemon

My obsession with za'atar continues with this simple and satisfying dish. The combination of sesame seeds, oregano, and thyme in za'atar pairs perfectly with avocado and lemon. I like to sprinkle on a little paprika for extra spice, but you could also use red chile flakes if you prefer.

Serves 2

1. Cut the avocado in half lengthwise and remove the pit.

2. Drizzle each half with a teaspoon of olive oil.

3. Sprinkle the za'atar, paprika, sea salt, and lemon zest on each half.

4. Serve a half avocado per person.

ASIA

INGREDIENTS

1 ripe avocado

2 tablespoons crumbled nori seaweed

2 teaspoons sesame salt (gomasio)

Drizzle of Asian-Style Dressing (optional) (page 166)

2 tablespoons sliced scallions

This dish combines several superfoods: seaweed, sesame, and avocado. And it's straight-up delicious. Gomasio is a seasoning made with salt and sesame seeds—you can find it at Asian markets or online, or you can make your own by pulsing two tablespoons of roasted sesame seeds with one teaspoon of salt in a spice grinder.

Serves 2

1. Cut the avocado in half lengthwise and remove the pit.

2. Sprinkle each half with nori and sesame salt, and top with a drizzle of dressing, if using.

3. Sprinkle with the scallions and serve a half avocado per person.

SWEET POTATOES

Sweet potatoes are a delicious, versatile, and inexpensive complex carb. They're packed with vitamins A and C, along with beta-carotene, which helps protect your skin from UV damage. Sweet potatoes are also high in gut-friendly fiber and score lower on the glycemic index than regular white potatoes (so they won't cause a blood sugar spike). Here are three ways to enjoy them: whipped, as fries, or baked and fully loaded.

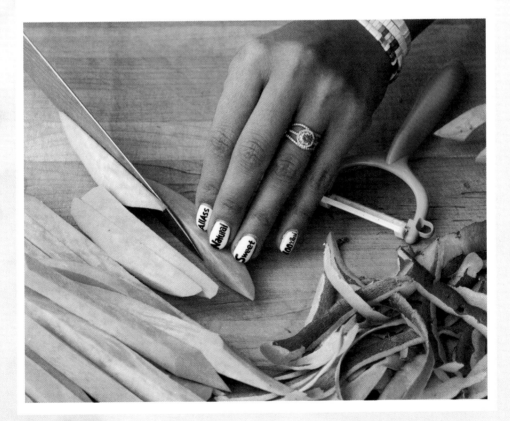

WHIPPED SWEET POTATOES

INGREDIENTS

2 cups diced peeled sweet potatoes (about 2 large)

1 cup chicken bone broth (see page 127) or water, plus more as needed

1 vanilla bean, seeds scraped (optional)

Finely grated zest and juice of 1 orange

2 tablespoons unsalted butter or coconut cream

$\frac{1}{2}$ teaspoon ground cinnamon

1 teaspoon paprika

$\frac{1}{4}$ teaspoon ground cumin

1 teaspoon salt, or more as needed

The silky-smooth texture of these whipped potatoes is a such a great alternative to the classic mashed potato. It's a little more work, but worth it! I like to whip these up (haha) when I'm cooking for a gathering that feels a little more formal.

Serves 4

1. Place the sweet potatoes and broth in a covered saucepan. Add the vanilla bean, if using, and orange zest.

2. Cook, covered, on medium heat, adding liquid as needed so the pan doesn't go dry.

3. When the potatoes are tender, add the orange juice and butter and whisk until smooth.

4. Add the cinnamon, paprika, cumin, and salt. Whisk to combine, then taste. Adjust the seasonings to your taste and serve.

do
what
feels
good

LOADED SWEET POTATOES

I like to think of this dish as the perfect pub food because it's jammed with everything except crappy ingredients and too much oil. It's also a super-versatile idea—you can easily sub out an ingredient and add in some others. If you want to make it vegan, just ditch the bacon and dairy cheese; I make it that way all the time, and sometimes I also like to add black olives and jalapeños.

Serves 4

1. Preheat the oven to 400°F. Pierce the sweet potatoes with the tines of a fork and rub them with the avocado oil. Bake until tender, 35 to 40 minutes.

2. Meanwhile, cook the bacon in a large skillet over medium-high heat. When the bacon is crisp and the fat has rendered, carefully remove it from the pan with a slotted spoon, reserving the fat in the pan.

3. Add the onion and broccoli to the pan along with ½ teaspoon of the salt and cook over medium heat until the broccoli has cooked through and the onions are tender.

4. Add the garlic and cook an additional minute until fragrant. Set aside.

5. When the potatoes are baked, split them in half lengthwise, and carefully scoop the cooked potato into a bowl. Reserve the skins. Add the remaining ½ teaspoon salt, coconut cream, paprika, and cinnamon.

6. Carefully scoop the mixture back into the reserved potato skins, and top with the cheese. Put back in the oven and bake for 5 minutes more, or until the cheese has melted.

7. Top with the chives and serve.

4 small sweet potatoes

2 teaspoons avocado oil

4 strips bacon, thinly sliced

1 onion, diced

2 cups broccoli florets, diced

1 teaspoon sea salt

2 garlic cloves, minced

4 tablespoons coconut cream

$\frac{1}{2}$ teaspoon smoked paprika (or chipotle powder, if you like a kick)

$\frac{1}{4}$ teaspoon ground cinnamon

$\frac{1}{4}$ cup shredded sharp cheddar (or goat's milk cheddar)

$\frac{1}{4}$ cup finely chopped chives or scallions

SWEET POTATO FRIES

INGREDIENTS

2 pounds sweet potatoes, peeled and cut into skinny French-fry shapes

2 tablespoons avocado oil

1 teaspoon garlic powder

1 teaspoon paprika

1 teaspoon salt

$\frac{1}{2}$ teaspoon ground cinnamon

$\frac{1}{2}$ teaspoon freshly ground black pepper

Green Goddess Dressing (page 168)

These are the guilt-free fries you've been looking for! I love this recipe because it makes a good amount of fries, so I'll have leftovers. These fries can be dipped into just about everything, but I love them with my Green Goddess Dressing on page 168.

Serves 4

1. Preheat the oven to 450°F. Place a baking sheet inside the oven as it preheats (for crispier fries).

2. In a large bowl, toss the sweet potatoes with the avocado oil until thoroughly coated.

3. In a small bowl, mix the garlic powder, paprika, salt, cinnamon, and black pepper. Pour into a clean paper bag.

4. Add the sweet potatoes and shake to thoroughly coat.

5. Transfer the sweet potatoes to the hot baking sheet and spread out in a single even layer.

6. Bake on the top shelf of the oven for 7 to 8 minutes, then turn the potatoes over and bake for another 8 minutes.

7. Serve with the Green Goddess Dressing, for dipping.

do
what
feels
good

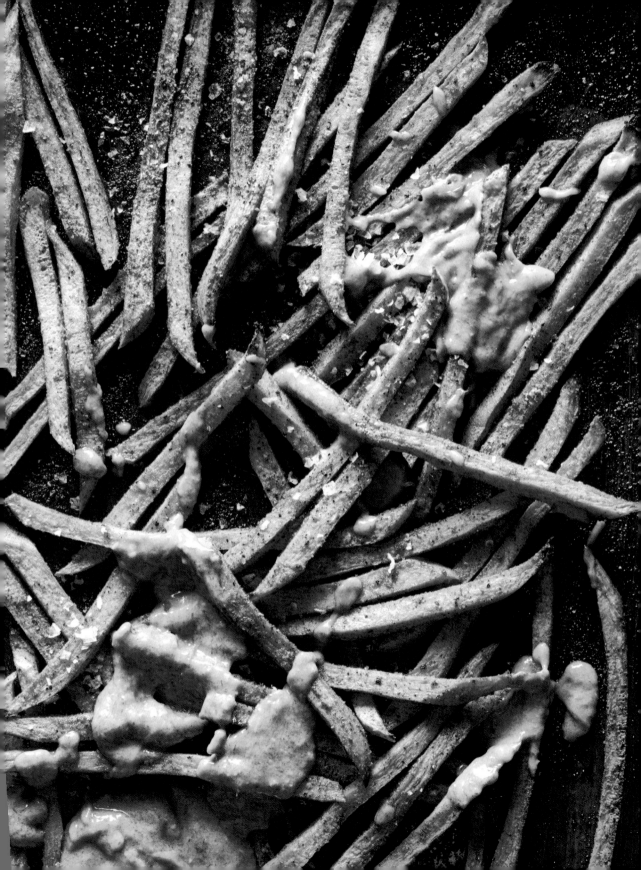

CAULIFLOWER

I've become a big fan of cauliflower recently. I love how versatile it is—you can slice a whole stalk into "steaks" and roast them; chop up the florets finely for healthier "rice" to use as a base for any variety of dishes, and even substitute it for flour in pizza dough (I know it sounds weird, but it makes a crust that is crispy and delicious!). Cauliflower is a cruciferous vegetable (its cousins include Brussels sprouts, cabbage, arugula, and kale), which means it contains prebiotic fiber that your gut bacteria need to stay healthy and keep you healthy. A serving of cauliflower also contains an entire day's worth of your recommended vitamin C intake! That's a lot to love in a simple, humble vegetable.

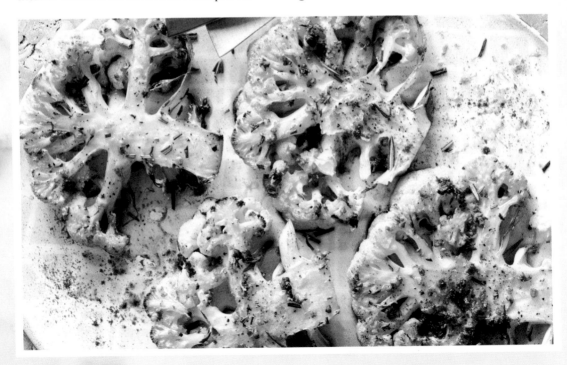

CAULIFLOWER STEAKS

When I was in Tel Aviv, I had one of the best whole roasted cauliflowers I've ever eaten. I was intimidated by roasting the entire thing at home, so I opted for an easier approach: cutting the cauliflower into "steaks" and roasting them. These steaks come out beautifully and are ideal for a dinner party.

Serves 4

1. Preheat the oven to 400°F. Line a baking sheet with parchment paper. Set aside.

2. Cut the cauliflower lengthwise through the core into 4 equal-size steaks and arrange on the baking sheet.

3. Whisk together the oil, lemon zest and juice, cayenne, garlic, and rosemary.

4. Brush half the mixture on top of the steaks and bake for 15 to 20 minutes, until the tops are golden brown.

5. Flip the steaks over, and brush with the remaining oil mixture. Bake an additional 10 to 15 minutes, until tender and golden brown.

INGREDIENTS

1 head cauliflower

$\frac{1}{4}$ cup olive oil

Finely grated zest and juice of 1 lemon

$\frac{1}{2}$ teaspoon cayenne pepper

3 garlic cloves, minced

$\frac{1}{4}$ cup fresh rosemary, minced

CAULIFLOWER PIZZA

INGREDIENTS

FOR THE SAUCE

1 tablespoon extra-virgin olive oil

1 small yellow onion, diced

3 garlic cloves, minced

1 teaspoon sea salt

1 teaspoon dried basil

1 teaspoon paprika

1 teaspoon freshly ground black pepper

1 (28-ounce) can crushed tomatoes

How many times have you seen something clever and you think to yourself, "How did I not come up with that??" Cauliflower pizza crust is one of those things! This nutrient-dense pizza crust is such a fabulous alternative to regular old flour crust and you still get the best flavors from the thousand different ways you can top this bad boy.

Makes one 8- to 10-inch pizza; serves 4

MAKE THE SAUCE

1. Heat the oil in a medium saucepan over medium-high heat. Add the onion and sauté, stirring frequently, until the onion is tender.

2. Add the garlic, salt, basil, paprika, and pepper and cook an additional 2 to 3 minutes, until fragrant.

3. Add the tomatoes, reduce the heat to low, and simmer until thickened, 30 to 40 minutes.

4. If you like a chunky sauce, leave as is, or blend for a smooth sauce.

5. Store for up to 1 week in the refrigerator, or up to 6 months in the freezer.

MAKE THE CRUST

1. Preheat the oven to 425°F. Line a baking sheet with parchment paper and set aside.

2. In a food processor, pulse the cauliflower into a fine powder.

3. Transfer to a pot with about ¼ cup of water and steam until tender.

4. Remove from the heat, transfer to a dry kitchen towel, and allow to cool.

5. Gather the ends of the towel and squeeze out any excess liquid until the cauliflower is dry.

6. Add the cauliflower to a bowl, along with the remaining crust ingredients, and stir to combine.

*do
what
feels
good*

7. Pour the mixture onto the prepared baking sheet and pat into a 10- to 12-inch circle.

8. Bake until golden brown, 10 to 15 minutes, then remove from the oven and top with the sauce and toppings as desired.

9. Bake for 10 minutes more and serve hot!

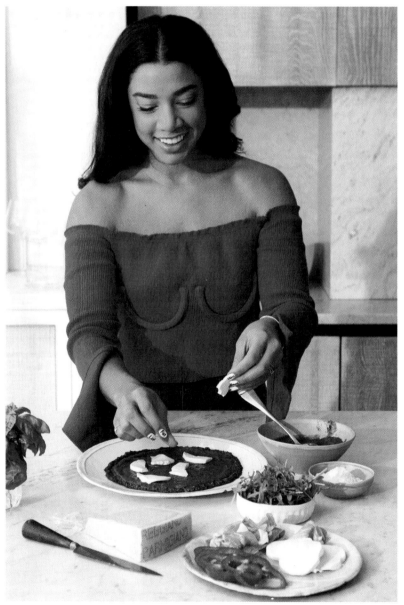

FOR THE CRUST

1 medium head of cauliflower, leaves and core removed

2 large eggs

$\frac{1}{4}$ cup Parmesan cheese

$\frac{1}{2}$ teaspoon garlic powder

$\frac{1}{2}$ teaspoon dried oregano

$\frac{1}{4}$ teaspoon paprika

OPTIONAL TOPPINGS

$\frac{1}{4}$ cup tomato sauce (recipe above)

$\frac{1}{4}$ cup pesto (instead of sauce or with it)

$\frac{1}{2}$ cup shredded cheese such as mozzarella

2 ounces prosciutto, pepperoni, or cooked sausage

1 cup chopped veggies (peppers, onions, broccoli, spinach, and zucchini are favorites)

Fresh greens, such as arugula or basil

CAULIFLOWER RICE

INGREDIENTS

1 head cauliflower, leaves and core removed

$\frac{1}{4}$ cup extra-virgin olive oil

1 yellow onion, diced

$\frac{1}{2}$ teaspoon sea salt

$\frac{1}{2}$ teaspoon ground white pepper

Cauliflower rice can be used just like regular rice. It makes a nice foundation for a bowl with veggies and protein and works well in stir-fries. Heck, you could even wrap it up in a nori sheet for some hand-made sushi! I suggest making a big batch and stashing some in the freezer for quick, easy meals on the fly.

Serves 4

1. In a food processor, pulse the cauliflower into rice-size bits (about 20 pulses).

2. Heat the oil in a large sauté pan. Add the onion and cook until tender.

3. Add the cauliflower rice, salt, and white pepper and cook, stirring frequently, for 5 to 10 minutes, then serve.

4. Store leftovers in the refrigerator for 3 to 5 days. Reheat with a little oil on the stovetop before serving.

RICE TO RICHES

Once you've got yourself a nice big batch of cauliflower rice, the possibilities for quick, easy meals are endless. Here are a few of my favorite combinations.

cauliflower fried rice: Sauté rice with ginger, garlic, and scallions, and season with a few splashes of coconut aminos or tamari sauce. Scramble an egg in when hot.

cauliflower risotto: Cook the rice as instructed, then add ¼ cup of white wine. Cook until evaporated, then fold in ½ cup Parmesan cheese and the zest of 1 lemon.

cilantro lime rice: Cook the rice as instructed, then fold in the zest and juice of 1 lime, ½ teaspoon of ground cumin, and ¼ cup of minced cilantro.

SALMON

It's a good thing salmon is super healthy because it is legit one of my favorite foods. I've already discussed my love of smoked salmon, but the infatuation doesn't stop there. The amazing thing is that different cooking methods really bring out different flavors and textures in the fish. I've included some of my favorite preparations here—salt-cured, baked, poached, and grilled. No matter how you prepare it, this beautiful fish is full of omega-3 fats that are great for your heart, your brain, and your skin.

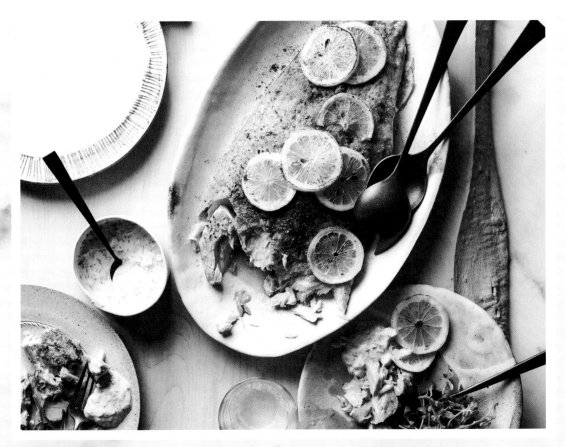

SALT-CURED SALMON

INGREDIENTS

3 to 4 salmon fillets, skin on

2 red beets, peeled

Finely grated zest of 1 lemon

Finely grated zest of
1 orange

$\frac{1}{3}$ cup sea salt

$\frac{1}{4}$ cup raw muscovado sugar

$\frac{1}{4}$ cup minced fresh dill

$\frac{1}{4}$ cup minced fresh tarragon

1 cup cream cheese or
coconut yogurt, for serving

Growing up a Jewish girl in New York, my love of smoked salmon runs deep. I always got my salmon at Jewish delis, like my personal fave Russ and Daughters, but I recently learned how to quick-cure it at home. My friends, who opened an amazing bagel store called Black Seed Bagels, taught me how to do it, and now I'm hooked. I feel like my grandpa is proud of me for this one!

Serves 4 to 8

1. Carefully remove any pin bones from the salmon, using a tweezer or a set of pliers. Place the salmon on a baking sheet, skin side down.

2. Using a box grater, grate the beets into a large bowl.

3. Add the lemon and orange zests, along with the salt, sugar, dill, and tarragon.

4. Using a spoon or a spatula, carefully pack the beet mixture onto the salmon.

5. Carefully wrap the salmon in wax paper or parchment paper, and then in plastic wrap, allowing it as little air as possible.

6. Cure in the refrigerator for 24 hours, then carefully rinse the salmon.

7. Serve thinly sliced, with the cream cheese.

do
what
feels
good

SPICE-RUBBED SALMON WITH CUCUMBER-YOGURT SAUCE

When I was a kid, my mother loved to make a salmon steak. But hers were always covered in garlic, and I swear I would smell garlic on her for at least 24 hours after she ate it. Definitely one of her anti-aging secrets, but not a great way to make new friends! My version, which uses just a little garlic powder, will leave you smelling fresh. The lemon-cucumber-herb yogurt sauce, a jazzed-up version of tzatziki, really makes this dish special.

Makes 4 generous servings

1. Preheat the oven to 375°F. Lightly oil a shallow baking dish with half the olive oil and set the salmon steaks in the dish. Drizzle the remaining oil over the top of the salmon.

2. In a small bowl, combine the orange and lemon zests, garlic, paprika, sea salt, black pepper, and cinnamon.

3. When well combined, pat onto both sides of the salmon.

4. Top the salmon with the lemon slices (they add flavor and protect the spices from burning), and bake, uncovered, for about 20 minutes.

5. While the salmon is baking, make the sauce: Put all the sauce ingredients in a small bowl and whisk together until well combined. Taste, and season with salt as needed.

6. Serve the salmon steaks with about ¼ cup of herb sauce per serving.

INGREDIENTS

FOR THE SALMON

$\frac{1}{4}$ cup olive oil

4 salmon steaks, skin on

Finely grated zest of 1 orange

Finely grated zest of 1 lemon

1 teaspoon powdered garlic

1 teaspoon paprika

1 teaspoon sea salt

1 teaspoon freshly ground black pepper

$\frac{1}{2}$ teaspoon ground cinnamon

1 lemon, sliced (the one you zested is perfect, see above)

FOR THE SAUCE

1 cup plain Greek yogurt or plain coconut yogurt

Juice of 1 lemon

$\frac{1}{4}$ cup minced fresh dill

$\frac{1}{4}$ cup minced fresh mint

$\frac{1}{4}$ cup minced fresh flat-leaf parsley

1 shallot, minced

1 Persian cucumber, peeled and diced (about $\frac{1}{2}$ cup)

Salt

POACHED SALMON SALAD

INGREDIENTS

FOR THE SALMON

1 (1-pound) salmon fillet, skin on

½ cup dry white wine (or ¼ cup lemon juice)

1 cup water

1 tablespoon sea salt

1 lemon, sliced

3 garlic cloves, sliced

4 sprigs fresh dill

FOR THE SALAD

1 recipe Green Goddess Dressing (page 168)

6 cups of your favorite greens

1 poached salmon fillet, at room temperature

1 red onion, thinly sliced

½ cup sliced green olives

1 red bell pepper, stemmed, seeded, and diced

1 mango, pitted, peeled, and diced

1 avocado, pitted, peeled, and diced

¼ cup chopped fresh dill

I love the simplicity of poached salmon. The poaching process retains the salmon's moisture and preserves its delicate, flaky texture. The fish becomes so soft that it literally falls apart when you cut into it, making it the perfect protein topping for a crisp green salad or a great option on sprouted grain toast or crackers.

Serves 4

FIRST, POACH THE SALMON

1. Remove the pin bones from the salmon and set the salmon aside.

2. In a large shallow pan, heat the wine, water, sea salt, lemon, garlic, and dill over low heat until the salt has dissolved.

3. Add the salmon and cook until firm, 10 to 15 minutes.

4. Serve warm, or at room temperature.

NEXT, ASSEMBLE THE SALAD

1. In a large salad bowl, toss together the dressing and greens until well combined. Top with the salmon, onion, olives, bell pepper, mango, and avocado.*

2. Sprinkle with the dill, and serve.

*You can also divide the dressed greens into individual salad bowls and make individual salads rather than one large shareable salad.

BRAISED CHICKEN

I love a nice, juicy piece of chicken and it is a go-to protein for me. But here's the thing: not all chicken is created equal. A lot of the chicken sold in this country is raised under pretty gross (and inhumane) conditions, which can make it a less-than-clean protein choice. So, if I'm going to eat chicken, I do my best to know where and how it was raised. I'm lucky to have a local halal butcher nearby, and I know they only sell chickens that were fed a real diet (i.e., not just grains and antibiotics) and were given access to run around and live as an animal should. Sometimes you can also find small farmers selling organic, humanely raised chickens at farmers' markets. If I have to buy my chicken at a grocery store, I always look for the word "pastured," which is a good sign that it was treated humanely and ate a healthy, well-rounded diet.

BRAISED LEMON CHICKEN

INGREDIENTS

1 whole chicken cut into 8 pieces, or 8 skin-on chicken thighs

1 teaspoon sea salt

$\frac{1}{4}$ cup extra-virgin olive oil

2 cups frozen artichoke hearts, thawed and patted dry*

$\frac{1}{4}$ cup finely minced fresh rosemary

Pinch of red chile flakes (optional)

10 garlic cloves, sliced

2 cups chicken bone broth (see page 127)

1 cup dry white wine

2 lemons, thinly sliced

"Braising" sounds like a fancy, difficult cooking technique, but I swear it's not. It basically just means that you're cooking the meat in liquid after first cooking it over high heat to get a nice crispy texture on the outside. This recipe is one of my absolute favorites. The combination of rosemary, lemon, and artichokes is delicious, comforting, and deeply satisfying.

Serves 4 to 8

1. Preheat the oven to 350°F. Sprinkle the chicken with the salt.

2. Heat a large oven-safe skillet or Dutch oven with a tight-fitting lid over medium-high heat.

3. While the skillet is heating, pat the chicken dry.

4. Add the oil to the skillet, then add the chicken, skin side down.

5. Cook for 5 to 10 minutes, or until the skin is golden brown and crisp.

6. Remove the skillet from the heat and transfer the chicken to a plate. Add the artichoke hearts, rosemary, chile flakes, and garlic to the skillet. Cook until the artichoke hearts are golden brown.

7. Return the chicken to the skillet, skin side up, along with the broth, wine, and lemons.

8. Cover the skillet and transfer to the oven. Cook for 30 to 35 minutes, or until the chicken is tender.

9. Remove the lid, and cook for an additional 10 minutes, to re-crisp the skin before serving. Serve immediately.

10. Leftovers can be stored in an airtight container in the fridge for up to 5 days.

*If you can't find frozen artichoke hearts, use low-sodium canned ones—just rinse and dry them really well before serving.

do
what
feels
good

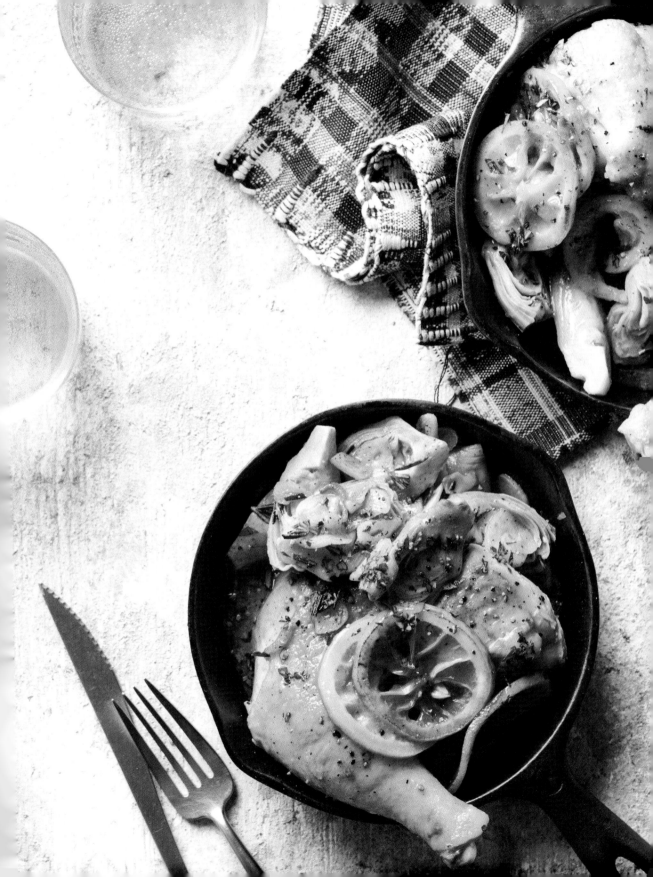

BRAISED CHIPOTLE CHICKEN

FOR THE MOLE SAUCE

3 tablespoons avocado oil

½ large yellow onion, minced

8 garlic cloves, diced

1 tablespoon whole cumin seeds

1 tablespoon whole coriander seeds

1 tablespoon dried oregano

1 can chipotles in adobo sauce*

Finely grated zest and juice of 1 orange

½ cup raisins

3 ounces bittersweet chocolate, diced

½ cup pumpkin seeds

1 cups chicken bone broth (see page 127)

1 cup full-fat coconut milk (or more to tame the heat)

½ teaspoon sea salt

This Mexican-inspired dish is crazy good, and the meat will last you for days. Pair it with cauliflower rice or tuck it into tortillas to make chicken tacos for quick weeknight meals. You will not regret putting in the extra effort with all of the spices—the result is well worth it.

Serves 6

FIRST, MAKE THE MOLE SAUCE

1. Heat the avocado oil in a large saucepan over medium heat.

2. Add the onion, garlic, and cumin and coriander seeds and cook, stirring occasionally, until the onion is tender, the spices are toasted, and the whole mixture is very fragrant.

3. Add the oregano, and cook for 1 minute more, then add the chipotles, orange zest, and raisins.

4. Cook for 2 to 3 minutes, then add the chocolate, pumpkin seeds, broth, coconut milk, and orange juice. Stir until the chocolate has melted.

5. Let simmer for 15 to 20 minutes, then transfer to a blender** and blend until smooth.

6. Return to the saucepan, add the salt, bring to a simmer, and let simmer, covered, for 10 to 15 minutes more.

*If you really struggle with spicy food, start with ¼ to ½ of a can.

**If you have an immersion blender, feel free to use that right in the pot, instead of transferring to a blender and back again.

*do
what
feels
good*

NEXT, PREPARE THE DISH

1. Preheat the oven to 350°F.

2. In a large oven-safe skillet with a lid, heat the avocado oil over medium-high heat.

3. Salt the chicken, add to the skillet, and cook, skin side down, until the skin is very crispy.

4. Flip the chicken and add the mole sauce to the skillet. Cover, transfer to the oven, and bake for 30 to 35 minutes.

5. Uncover, and continue to bake for 10 minutes more.

6. Serve immediately topped with the mango, onion, cilantro, and sesame seeds.

7. Leftovers can be stored in an airtight container in the fridge for up to 5 days. Be aware that the spices in the dish develop as it rests, so it may be spicier the next day.

FOR THE CHICKEN

1 tablespoon avocado oil

1 teaspoon sea salt

8 chicken thighs, or 1 whole chicken cut into 8 pieces

1 ripe mango, minced

$\frac{1}{2}$ red onion, minced

$\frac{1}{2}$ cup fresh cilantro, minced

$\frac{1}{4}$ cup toasted sesame seeds

BRAISED CHICKEN WITH APRICOT AND OLIVES

INGREDIENTS

8 chicken thighs, or 1 chicken cut into 8 pieces

1 teaspoon sea salt

$\frac{1}{4}$ cup extra-virgin olive oil

1 white onion, roughly chopped

1 fennel bulb, trimmed and roughly chopped

1 cup unsweetened dried apricots, roughly chopped

1 teaspoon ground ginger

1 teaspoon ground cumin

$\frac{1}{4}$ teaspoon ground cinnamon

1 teaspoon freshly ground black pepper

Finely grated zest and juice of 1 orange

2 cups chicken bone broth (see page 127)

1 cup pitted green olives

This recipe is sweet and tangy and reminds me a lot of the tagine cooking of Morocco, where Brendan and I got married. We were blown away by the cuisine in North Africa. I created this recipe after we came home from our trip, and every time I make it I am reminded of our magical time there.

Serves 4 to 8

1. Preheat the oven to 350°F. Sprinkle the chicken with the salt.

2. Heat a large oven-safe skillet or Dutch oven with a tight-fitting lid over medium-high heat.

3. While the skillet is heating, pat the chicken dry.

4. Add the oil to the pan, then add the chicken, skin side down.

5. Cook for 5 to 10 minutes, or until the skin is golden brown and crisp.

6. Remove the chicken from the skillet and set aside.

7. Add the onion, fennel, apricots, ginger, cumin, cinnamon, black pepper, and the orange zest to the skillet. Cook, stirring occasionally, until the onion and fennel are tender.

8. Return the chicken to the skillet and add the orange juice and chicken broth. Cook, covered, for 35 minutes, or until the chicken is tender.

9. Remove the lid, add the olives, and cook for an additional 10 to 15 minutes to re-crisp the skin. Serve immediately.

10. Leftovers can be stored in an airtight container in the fridge for up to 5 days.

do
what
feels
good

PARMESAN FOR ALL

Parmesan cheese—real Parmesan—is an important staple of any cook's pantry. It packs such a salty, nutty punch of flavor that just a sprinkle can really enhance a dish. It pairs well with so many foods—from tomatoes to chicken to eggs to veggies. Of course, my introduction to Parmesan was in New York City. Every pizza place has an eggplant Parmesan and a chicken Parmesan that you can order as a sandwich, heaped on a roll with extra mozzarella, or as a platter, with pasta on the side. I'm partial to an open-faced platter situation, which was the inspiration for these recipes. My remakes are decidedly less greasy than the originals, but they're just as satisfying.

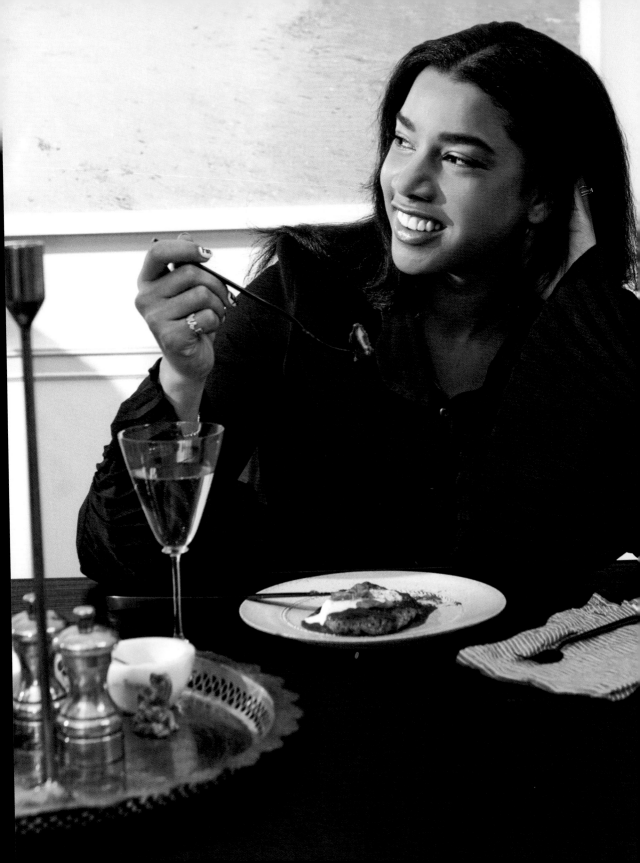

CHICKEN PARMESAN

Sometimes you just want chicken Parm. If you're going to go there, I say, why not make it yourself with the freshest ingredients possible? This classic Italian dish is great for a group and is super kid-friendly. If you've avoiding dairy, you can use vegan mozzarella, but I suggest splurging on the Parm, if you can.

Serves 4

1. If using chicken breasts, carefully split each one in half as if you were butterflying it, to create two equal size cutlets from each breast.

2. Using a rolling pin, pound the chicken thin, between sheets of plastic wrap, until ¼ or ½ inch thickness.

3. Sprinkle with the salt and set aside.

4. Meanwhile, whisk the eggs in a small bowl or pie dish and set aside.

5. In another bowl or pie dish, whisk together the almonds, Parmesan cheese, basil, paprika, garlic, and oregano. Set aside.

6. Pat the chicken cutlets dry with a paper towel, then toss in the tapioca starch to coat.

7. Transfer the cutlets to the egg mixture, and then to almond mixture to bread.

8. Heat a large skillet over medium-high heat. When hot, add the oil. Add the breaded cutlets and sear for 3 to 4 minutes per side until golden brown and crispy.

9. Reduce the heat to low. Add the tomato sauce and simmer for 5 to 10 minutes.

10. Top the cutlets with the mozzarella and continue to cook until the cheese has melted. Serve immediately.

INGREDIENTS

2 boneless, skinless chicken breasts (or 4 chicken cutlets)

1 teaspoon sea salt

2 large eggs

¾ cup ground almonds

¼ cup grated Parmesan cheese

1 teaspoon dried basil

1 teaspoon paprika

1 teaspoon garlic powder

1 teaspoon dried oregano

½ cup tapioca starch

¼ cup extra-virgin olive oil

3 cups tomato sauce (see sauce recipe for Cauliflower Pizza, page 180)

1 cup shredded mozzarella cheese (or vegan cheese)

EGGPLANT PARMESAN

INGREDIENTS

2 tablespoons olive oil

1 large eggplant

1 teaspoon sea salt

2 large eggs

¾ cup ground almonds

¼ cup grated Parmesan cheese

1 teaspoon dried basil

1 teaspoon paprika

1 teaspoon garlic powder

1 teaspoon dried oregano

3 cups tomato sauce (see sauce recipe for Cauliflower Pizza, page 180)

1 cup shredded mozzarella cheese

This was one of the first dishes Brendan and I shared when we started dating. We went to Lil' Frankies in the East Village and split the eggplant Parm. We love this dish and make it at home when we feel like reminiscing. I love the flavor and texture combo, and I think you will, too.

Serves 4

1. Preheat the oven to 400°F. Grease a baking sheet with the oil and set aside.

2. Remove the stem end from the eggplant and slice the eggplant into ½-inch rounds. Salt them thoroughly and set on a clean kitchen towel. Leave for 15 to 20 minutes, to draw out the moisture.

3. Meanwhile, whisk the eggs in a small bowl or pie dish and set aside.

4. In another bowl or pie dish, whisk together the almonds, Parmesan cheese, basil, paprika, garlic, and oregano. Set aside.

5. Brush the salt from the eggplant and press the slices with a towel to draw out any excess moisture.

6. Dip the eggplant slices in the egg mixture, then in the almond mixture, and transfer to a baking sheet.

7. Bake for 15 to 20 minutes, then turn carefully, and continue to bake until golden brown and crispy

8. Spoon the tomato sauce onto the baking sheet (around and on top of the eggplant) and top each round with the mozzarella cheese.

9. Return to the oven and bake for 5 to 10 minutes, until the sauce is hot and the cheese has melted. Serve immediately.

do
what
feels
good

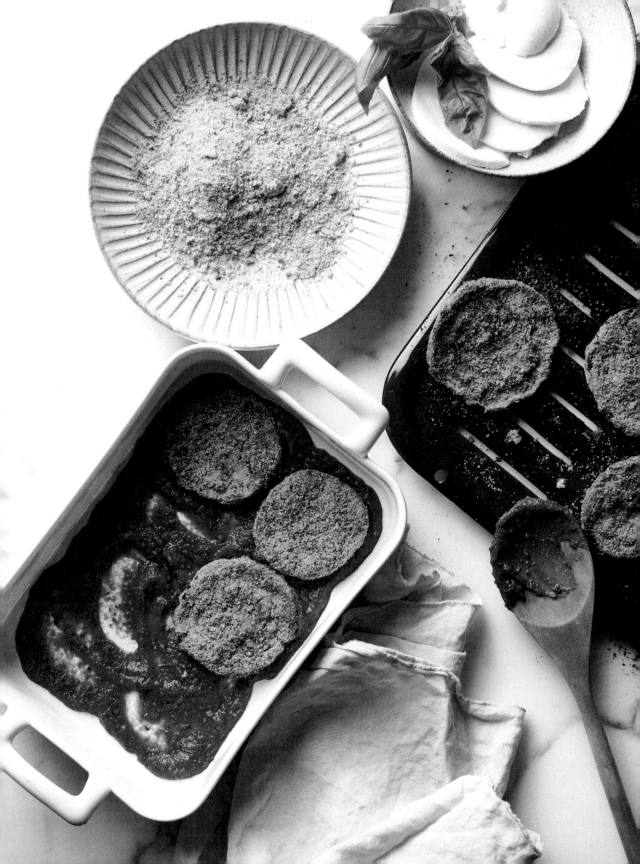

VEGAN "PARM"

INGREDIENTS

2 tablespoons extra-virgin olive oil

4 medium zucchini

1 teaspoon sea salt

$\frac{3}{4}$ cup ground almonds

$\frac{1}{4}$ cup nutritional yeast

1 teaspoon dried basil

1 teaspoon paprika

1 teaspoon garlic powder

1 teaspoon dried oregano

1–2 tablespoons Dijon mustard

3 cups tomato sauce (see sauce recipe for Cauliflower Pizza, page 180)

1 cup cashew cheese (see page 143) or shredded vegan mozzarella

This dish is packed with protein and nutrients and makes for a delish vegan alternative to regular Parm. Other than the zucchini as a stand-in for chicken, you'll hardly notice a difference in taste thanks to the star ingredient, nutritional yeast, which is my absolute favorite cheesy alternative to dairy cheese.

Serves 4

1. Preheat the oven to 400°F. Grease a baking sheet with the oil and set aside.

2. Remove the stem end from the zucchini and slice them into ½-inch slices, lengthwise. Salt the slices thoroughly and set on a clean kitchen towel. Leave for 15 to 20 minutes, to draw out the moisture.

3. Whisk together the almonds, nutritional yeast, basil, paprika, garlic, and oregano. Set aside.

4. Brush the salt from the zucchini and press the slices with a towel to draw out any excess moisture.

5. Brush the slices with a thin coating of mustard on each side, then roll in the almond mixture.

6. Transfer to the prepared baking sheet and bake for 15 to 20 minutes. Flip carefully and continue to bake until golden brown and crispy.

7. Spoon the tomato sauce onto the baking sheet (around and on top of the zucchini) and top each slice with a dollop of cashew cheese.

8. Return to the oven and bake for 5 to 10 minutes more. Serve immediately.

do
what
feels
good

ZUCCHINI NOODLES

Who doesn't love a noodle? They add heft and a satisfying slurp to any meal. Unfortunately, processed wheat noodles also add a dose of sugar and starch/gluten, which is not what I'm trying to eat most of the time. Enter the spiralizer and the miracle that is the zucchini noodle. Zoodles are one of my favorite sneaky ways to make sure I'm eating enough vegetables. They offer the same slurp factor as a traditional noodle and basically serve as a vehicle for sauce. I love a good rich sauce with my zoodles, and these three are my favorites.

TURKEY BOLOGNESE

INGREDIENTS

5 cups zucchini noodles
(about 4 medium zucchini)

1 teaspoon sea salt

$\frac{1}{4}$ cup extra-virgin olive oil

1 yellow onion, minced

1 pound ground turkey

4 garlic cloves, minced

Finely grated zest of 1 lemon

1 tablespoon dried basil

1 teaspoon garlic powder

1 teaspoon dried oregano

1 teaspoon fresh minced
rosemary

1 pound mushrooms,
finely diced

4 cups tomato sauce (see
sauce recipe for Cauliflower
Pizza, (page 180)

Bolognese is such a comfort food, and making it with ground turkey really lightens it up. You still get all the classic flavors, minus the food coma and bellyache. Seriously, there are few things I enjoy more than digging into a big bowl of saucy noodles, and this is one of my favorite ways to do so and still feel like a warrior afterward.

Serves 4

1. Add the zucchini noodles to a large bowl with ½ teaspoon of the salt and toss to combine. Set aside.

2. In a large stockpot, heat the olive oil over medium heat. Add the onion and the remaining ½ teaspoon salt and cook, stirring occasionally, until tender.

3. Add the turkey and cook until the turkey has browned and is cooked through, about 5 minutes.

4. Add the garlic, lemon zest, basil, garlic powder, oregano, and rosemary and cook until fragrant, 2 to 3 minutes.

5. Add the mushrooms and reduce the heat to low. Continue to cook until the veggies are tender, about 5 minutes. Add the tomato sauce, cover, and let simmer for 10 to 15 minutes.

6. Firmly pat the zucchini noodles dry, squeezing out the excess moisture.

7. Add the zucchini noodles to the sauce and increase the heat to medium-high. Cook for 2 to 3 minutes, until the zoodles are tender.

8. Serve as is, or top with grated Parmesan cheese and chopped fresh parsley.

do
what
feels
good

ITALIAN ZOODLES

I love pesto, and I like to play around with variations—different nuts, different herbs, different cheese. This spinach-walnut pesto is crazy good. You're going to want to make an extra batch just to have on hand for eggs, chicken, fish, or any dish that needs a little extra something.

Serves 4

1. In a large bowl, toss together the zucchini noodles and salt. Set aside.

2. Bring a large pot of water to a boil.

3. Place ½ cup of the walnuts along with the kale, spinach, and basil in a food processor or high-speed blender and pulse until combined.

4. Add the Parmesan cheese and lemon juice, and turn the food processor on low.

5. Stream in the olive oil to make a thick pesto. If too thick, add more oil, a teaspoon at a time.

6. When the water is boiling, add the zucchini noodles and cook until tender. Drain and transfer to a serving bowl.

7. Whisk ½ cup of the pesto with ½ cup of water, add to the zoodles, and toss.

8. Top with the lemon zest and the remaining toasted walnuts and serve.

INGREDIENTS

5 cups zucchini noodles (about 4 medium zucchini)

½ teaspoon sea salt

1 cup toasted walnuts

¼ cup fresh kale

¼ cup fresh baby spinach leaves

¼ cup fresh basil leaves

¼ cup grated Parmesan cheese or nutritional yeast

Juice of 1 lemon

¼ cup extra-virgin olive oil, give or take a tablespoon

Finely grated zest of 1 lemon

ZUCCHINI PAD THAI

INGREDIENTS

5 cups zucchini noodles
(about 4 medium zucchini)

½ teaspoon sea salt

Juice of 1 lime

2 tablespoons monk fruit
sweetener

2 tablespoons coconut
aminos

1 tablespoon fish sauce

1 tablespoon garlic chili
sauce (optional)

2 tablespoons sesame oil

1 tablespoon peeled and
minced fresh ginger

3 garlic cloves, minced

5 scallions, sliced, white and
green parts separated

1 red bell pepper, stemmed,
seeded, and diced

1 cup broccoli slaw

2 large eggs, lightly whisked

1 pound peeled and
deveined shrimp*

1 cup bean sprouts

¼ cup minced fresh cilantro

¼ cup finely minced cashews

1 lime, cut into wedges

Because I grew up in New York City and was raised by a single mom, takeout was a staple for me. Thai food has always been a favorite of mine, and pad thai is one of my weaknesses. This version offers the same great flavors and textures of the take-out classic but subs in zoodles for the noodles and cashews for the peanuts. The sauce is so good you may find yourself scooping it up with a spoon. No judgment here.

Serves 4

1. In a large bowl, toss together the zucchini noodles and salt. Set aside.

2. In a smaller bowl, whisk together the lime juice, monk fruit sweetener, coconut aminos, fish sauce, and garlic chili sauce, if using. Set aside.

3. Heat the sesame oil in a large sauté pan or wok. Add the ginger, garlic, and the white parts of the scallions. Cook for 2 to 3 minutes, then add the bell pepper and broccoli slaw.

4. Sauté for 2 to 3 minutes, stirring frequently, then add the eggs and shrimp and cook for 3 to 4 minutes more, until the eggs have scrambled and the shrimp have cooked through. The shrimp are ready when opaque and firm to the touch.

5. Firmly press the zoodles dry, and add to the pan, along with the reserved sauce. Cook until the zoodles are tender.

6. Serve topped with the bean sprouts, cilantro, cashews, and lime wedges.

*You can also skip the shrimp, or use cooked shredded chicken or cubed seitan, depending on your dietary preferences.

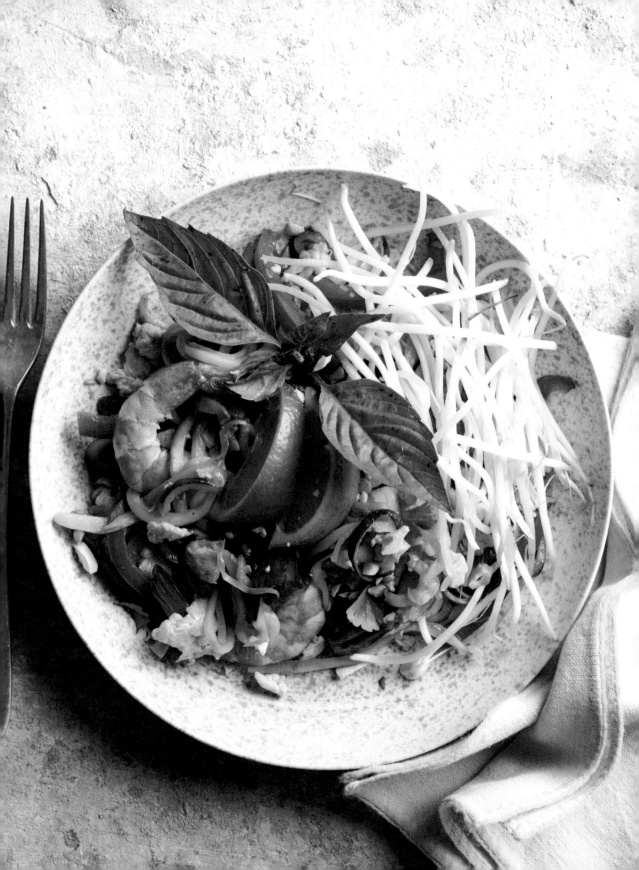

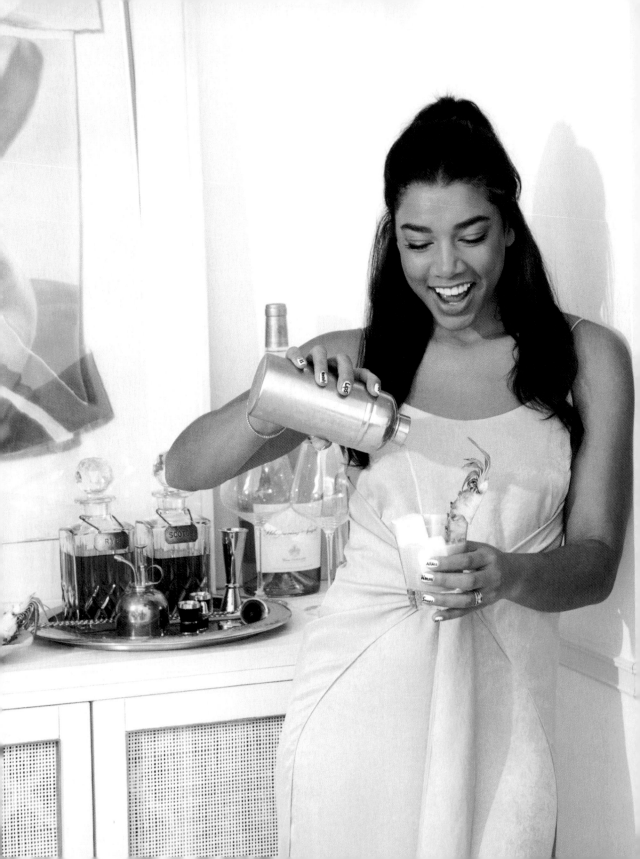

make it a DOUBLE

EVERYBODY'S ON THE COUCH GETTING TIPSY

TART CHERRY OLD-FASHIONED

INGREDIENTS

1 demerara sugar cube
or 1 teaspoon monk fruit
sweetener

2 to 3 dashes of orange or
Angostura bitters

1 ounce tart cherry juice,
such as Montmorency
cherry juice

Ice (ideally a single 2-inch
cube or sphere)

2 ounces bourbon

Strip of orange zest,
for garnish

Since 1881, people have been enjoying the combo of spirits, bitters, and sugar—maybe that's why the drink is called an Old-Fashioned. My version uses tart cherry juice, which is known to aid recovery for your muscles and adds a hit of antioxidants. It is also delicious.

Serves 1

1. Place the sugar in the bottom of a rocks glass and soak with the bitters.

2. Add the cherry juice and stir to dissolve the sugar.

3. Add the ice cube and bourbon, then garnish with the orange zest just before serving; give it a good squeeze to release the aromatics.

do
what
feels
good

JALISCO MULE

A mule is traditionally made with spirits and ginger beer. This one has a jalapeño, because I love some heat in a cocktail. Jalapeños contain capsaicin, which can help relieve pain and may even promote weight loss by boosting metabolism. The capsaicin is also what makes this drink delightfully spicy.

Serves 1

1. Fill a mule cup or highball glass with ice and set aside.

2. Muddle the jalapeño, if using, and the lime juice in the bottom of a cocktail shaker.

3. Add the tequila, coconut milk, ginger beer, and ice cubes and stir 10 to 15 seconds, until chilled.

4. Strain into the prepared cup, add the bitters, and serve garnished with the lime slice and candied ginger.

INGREDIENTS

1 slice jalapeño (optional)

Juice of $\frac{1}{2}$ lime

2 ounces tequila blanco

$\frac{1}{4}$ cup coconut milk

$\frac{1}{2}$ cup spicy ginger beer, such as Bundaberg

2 to 3 large ice cubes

2 dashes of Angostura bitters or grapefruit bitters

Lime slice, for garnish

Candied ginger, for garnish

TEQUILA

Tequila is one of my favorite spirits because it's low in carbs, doesn't spike your blood sugar, and mixes beautifully with spicy, sweet, and citrus flavors. And if you choose a tequila that is 100 percent agave, it will also contain a carbohydrate called fructan, which is actually a probiotic!

GOLDEN HOUR

2 ounces gin

1 tablespoon peeled and grated fresh turmeric or $\frac{1}{2}$ teaspoon ground dried turmeric

Juice of $\frac{1}{2}$ lime

4 ounces ginger beer

3 to 4 ice cubes

Candied ginger or turmeric, for garnish

Lime slice, for garnish

This mule relies on ginger beer as a base. I recommend looking for a brand that doesn't contain a ton of sugar—some ginger beers are super sweet. I use gin as the spirit and add fresh or dried turmeric for a beautiful golden hue and a little extra immune system support.

Serves 1

1. Add the gin, turmeric, lime juice, ginger beer, and ice cubes to a cocktail shaker.

2. Shake vigorously for 20 to 30 seconds, or until condensation appears on the shaker.

3. Strain into a rocks glass and garnish with the candied ginger and lime slice.

do
what
feels
good

CLASSIC CAESAR

When I first went to Canada and ordered a Bloody Mary, everyone looked at me like *Ohhhh, she's American!* The Caesar is Canada's Bloody Mary, and let me tell you the Canadian version is 100x better than an American Bloody and that is because they use Clamato juice instead of tomato juice. I know, I know, it looks a little sketchy, but it is delicious. Just trust.

Serves 1

1. Fill a glass with ice and set aside.
2. In a cocktail shaker, combine the celery salt, Clamato juice, vodka, horseradish, Worcestershire sauce, 1 ounce of pickle juice, and the black pepper.
3. Shake briefly to combine, then taste. Add the hot sauce and additional pickle juice as needed.
4. Pour into the glass, and garnish with your favorite option(s).

KICK IT UP

Before mixing the drink, rim the glass as follows: Run 1 lime wedge around the rim and then roll the glass in a mixture of 1 teaspoon of sea salt, 1 teaspoon of black pepper, and 1 teaspoon of smoked paprika. Pour the drink carefully into the rimmed glass.

INGREDIENTS

Ice

½ teaspoon celery salt

1 cup Clamato juice

2 ounces vodka

1 teaspoon grated horseradish (fresh or prepared)

½ teaspoon Worcestershire sauce

1 to 2 ounces pickle juice or lime juice

½ teaspoon freshly ground black pepper

Hot sauce

Celery stalk, pickle spears, olives, cocktail onions, fresh cilantro leaves, cooked pepper bacon, or pickled green beans, for garnish

BLUE MAGIC

INGREDIENTS

¼ cup passion fruit juice*

½ teaspoon agave nectar

¼ teaspoon Blue Majik algae powder

2 ounces aged light rum

1 once unsweetened coconut milk

2 to 3 dashes of orange or tiki bitters

1 cup ice cubes**

Fresh lime juice, as needed

Pineapple wedge, for garnish

My great-grandfather was a pioneer in the liquor business. Samuel Bronfman Sr. started out as a bootlegger in Canada during Prohibition and created a legacy that includes brands like Seagram's and Crown Royale. So it's no surprise I love a good cocktail, but I have a feeling my great-grandfather would be surprised to see this blue-hued beauty. I love a modern drink that combines an old-fashioned spirit with a healthy twist—here, in the form of Blue Majik, a kind of spirulina, which is great for fighting inflammation.

Serves 1

1. Place all the ingredients except the pineapple wedge in a blender and blend until smooth.

2. Taste, and add either additional agave or lime juice according to your preference.

3. Serve garnished with the pineapple wedge and, if desired, a few additional drops of bitters.

4. If you've got a cocktail umbrella—go for it!

*If you can't find passion fruit juice, use pineapple juice and skip the agave.

** For an even creamier cocktail, use frozen coconut meat, or a mixture of ice cubes and coconut meat.

do
what
feels
good

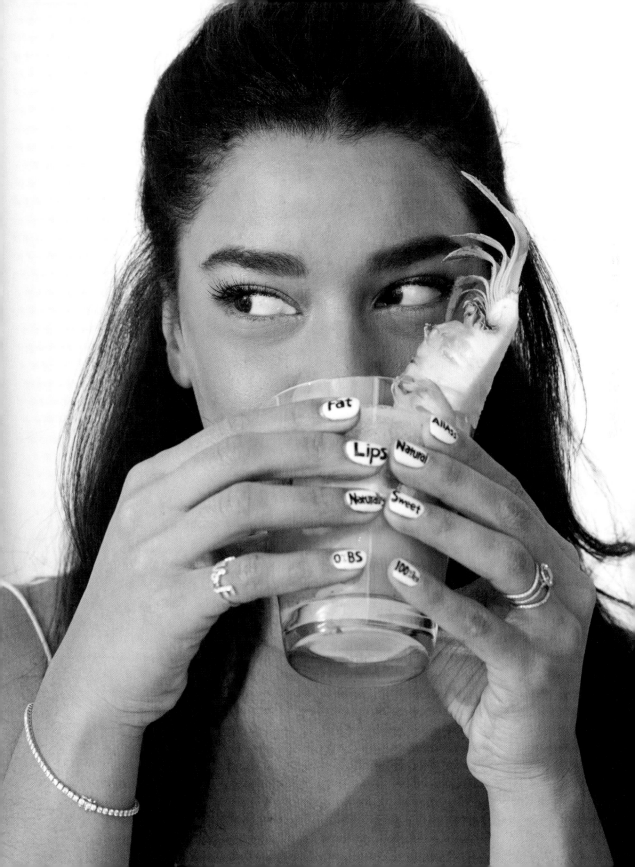

HOT HONEY

1–2 tablespoons raw honey

Juice of ½ lemon

½ cup boiling water

2 ounces bourbon

Dash of Angostura bitters (optional)

These cocktails are my twist on a hot toddy—a great drink when you have a sore throat, or when it's getting cold outside, or when you're curled up by a fire with a special someone. One basic recipe and five variations allows you to choose between spirits and flavors to keep your throat soothed, your hands warmed, and your soul happy.

Serves 1

1. Stir together the honey, lemon juice, and boiling water in a coffee mug until the honey is dissolved.

2. Add the bourbon and bitters, if using, and stir to combine.

3. Drink and enjoy.

VARIATIONS

GOLDEN TODDY: Add 1 tablespoon peeled and grated fresh turmeric when you add the honey and lemon juice to the glass.

JASMINE TODDY: Use ½ cup of hot jasmine tea instead of the boiling water, and swap the juice of 1 clementine for the lemon juice.

CANADIAN TODDY: Use Canadian whiskey instead of the bourbon, and sweeten with maple syrup instead of the honey.

EXTRA-HOT TODDY: Add ½ teaspoon cayenne pepper and a couple of slices of fresh ginger to the toddy when you add the honey and lemon juice to the mug.

CALIENTE TODDY: Make the hot toddy with mezcal instead of the bourbon, and lime juice instead of the lemon juice.

do
what
feels
good

SPARKLING ALOE

Aloe vera isn't the tastiest juice, but it's great for you—it helps with digestion and is super hydrating for your skin. In this refreshing cocktail, the bitterness of the aloe vera is masked by the muddled lime, cucumber, and basil. Mix it all up with some good-quality gin, and you've got a cocktail that is the perfect après-sun sip. (If you like your cocktails with some heat, muddle in a couple of jalapeño slices!)

Serves 1

1. Fill a highball glass with ice and set aside.

2. In a cocktail shaker, muddle together the basil, cucumber, lime juice, and stevia to taste.

3. Add the gin and aloe juice, along with the ice cubes, and shake vigorously for 10 to 15 seconds.

4. Strain into the highball glass, and top with the sparkling water.

5. Serve garnished with the cucumber slice.

INGREDIENTS

1 to 2 fresh basil leaves

1 cucumber slice

Juice of $\frac{1}{2}$ lime

5 to 6 drops liquid stevia

2 ounces cucumber-heavy gin, such as Hendrick's

2 ounces aloe vera juice

2 to 3 ice cubes

4 ounces sparkling water

1 cucumber slice, for garnish

BLACK ON BLACK/BLACK ON BLUE

INGREDIENTS

¼ cup blackberries or blueberries, plus more for garnish

1 small sprig thyme, plus more for garnish

2 ounces grapefruit juice (¼ to ½ of a grapefruit)

2 ounces black pepper vodka

2 to 3 ice cubes

4 to 6 drops liquid stevia, or as needed

2 ounces club soda

Black pepper, for garnish

Choose your own adventure with this sexy drink: Black pepper and blackberries, or black pepper and blueberries. Either version makes an eye-catching cocktail with a spicy kick. And black pepper is great for digestion, making this cocktail an excellent aperitif or post-dinner drink. You can buy infused black pepper vodka or make your own by pouring 2 tablespoons of whole black peppercorns into a 750-ml bottle of vodka. Let infuse in a cool dark place for 5 to 7 days, then use.

Serves 1

1. In a cocktail shaker, muddle the blackberries, thyme, and grapefruit juice together.

2. Add the black pepper vodka and the ice cubes and shake vigorously for 15 to 30 seconds.

3. Strain into a rocks glass and add the stevia and club soda.

4. Stir to combine, then taste and adjust to your preference; add more stevia for sweetness or additional grapefruit juice for tang.

5. Garnish with blackberries, thyme, and a grind of fresh pepper.

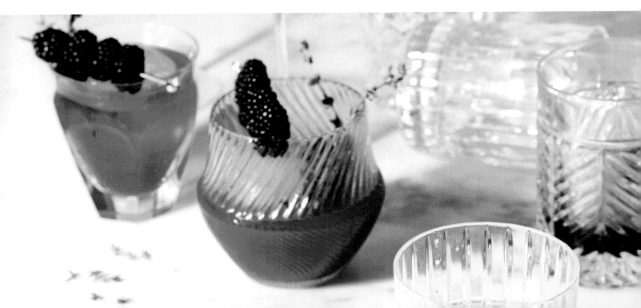

BLUE AGAVE

Margarita meets mule—gone blue. Tequila, pineapple, ginger beer, and Blue Majik combine for a delicious, refreshing cocktail. Ginger beer is wonderful if you're looking for some digestion support, so this is a good drink to have at a barbecue where you'll be eating all day.

Serves 1

1. Muddle together the tequila and pineapple in the bottom of a cocktail shaker.

2. Empty the contents of the Blue Magik capsule into the shaker, as well as the lime juice, tangerine juice, ginger beer, and stevia. Taste and adjust as needed.

3. Stir to combine, then add the ice cubes and stir until chilled, 10 to 15 seconds.

4. Strain into a rocks glass with ice, splash with bitters, and serve garnished with a lime wedge.

INGREDIENTS

2 ounces tequila

$\frac{1}{4}$ cup pineapple chunks

1 Blue Magik capsule

Juice of $\frac{1}{2}$ lime

Juice of 1 small tangerine, such as a clementine

4 ounces spicy ginger beer, such as Bundaberg

5 to 6 drops liquid stevia, or as needed

3 to 4 ice cubes

Dash of Angostura bitters

Lime wedge, for garnish

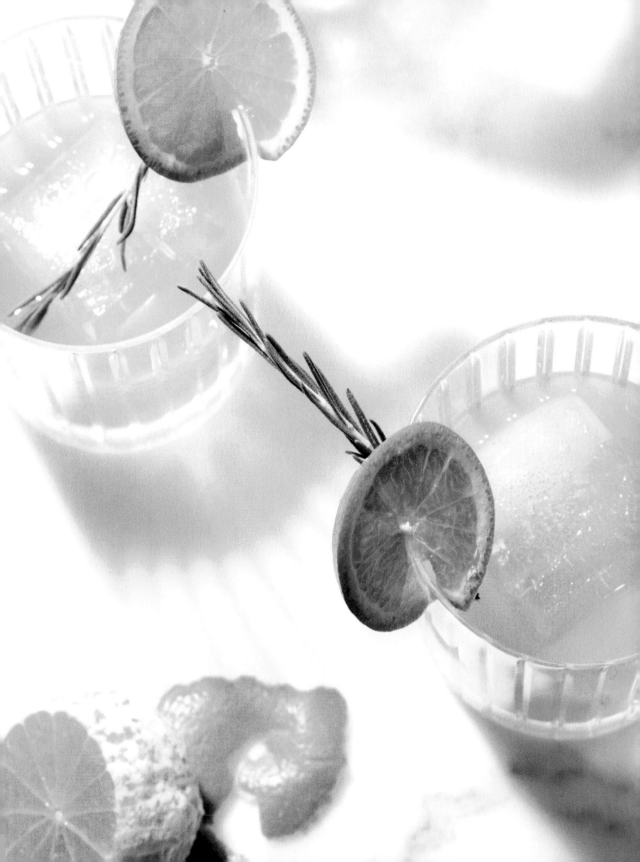

ONLY NONI

I first learned about noni in 2013 when I went to Australia, where I fell in love with all the fresh fruits and vegetables the climate had to offer. There was so much HEALTH going on there, especially in Byron Bay, where we stayed nearby on my aunt's biodynamic farm. Noni is a native superfood to the land down under, offering benefits like reducing inflammation, lowering cholesterol, and helping with cellular renewal. You can get noni online as a powder or a juice. This recipe uses the juice. If you can't source it, you can use pomegranate juice instead.

I came up with this cocktail using my favorite tequila, and if you like tequila as much as I do, then you'll welcome this new addition to your bar skills with open arms.

Serves 1

1. In the bottom of a cocktail shaker, muddle together the ginger, tangerine, and rosemary.

2. Add the tequila, agave, lime juice, and noni juice and taste.

3. Add more agave if needed, then add the ice cubes and shake vigorously for 30 seconds.

4. Strain into a rocks glass or champagne coupe and serve garnished with the tangerine wheel and sprig of rosemary.

INGREDIENTS

$1\frac{1}{2}$ teaspoons roughly chopped fresh ginger

$\frac{1}{4}$ small tangerine, such as a clementine

1 teaspoon fresh rosemary needles

2 ounces tequila blanco

1 teaspoon agave nectar

Juice of $\frac{1}{2}$ lime

2 ounces noni juice

3 to 4 ice cubes

1 tangerine wheel and 1 sprig rosemary, for garnish

AVORITA

INGREDIENTS

1 lime wedge, for the glass rim

1 tablespoon coarse salt

½ ripe avocado, pitted and peeled

1 cup ice

2 ounces good-quality tequila blanco

1 ounce Cointreau

Juice of 1 lime

1 to 2 teaspoons agave nectar

1 lime slice, for garnish

Sometimes I wish this cocktail was as ubiquitous as your basic avocado toast. Because as an aficionado of both avocados and fine tequilas, I feel like this cocktail was basically made for me, and me for it. Then there's the mango version—yes, the "avo-mango-rita," which is kind of like a nighttime smoothie. If you sometimes look longingly at frozen cocktails but you're wary of all that added sugar, this is definitely going to be your favorite summer jam.

Serves 1

1. Run the lime wedge around the rim of a margarita glass and roll it in the salt. Set aside.

2. Add the avocado, ice, tequila, Cointreau, lime juice, and ½ teaspoon of the agave to the blender and pulse until the ice is finely crushed.

3. Taste, and add more agave or lime juice as needed.

4. Serve in the salted glass, garnished with the lime slice.

KICK IT UP

Blend 1 to 2 slices of jalapeño into your drink and mix in some cayenne pepper with your salt before rimming the glass.

AVO-MANGO-RITA

Instead of the agave and Cointreau, blend in ¼ cup of mango chunks (frozen are fine). Serve garnished with mango and candied ginger. If using frozen mango, you can swap out some of the ice, too!

do
what
feels
good

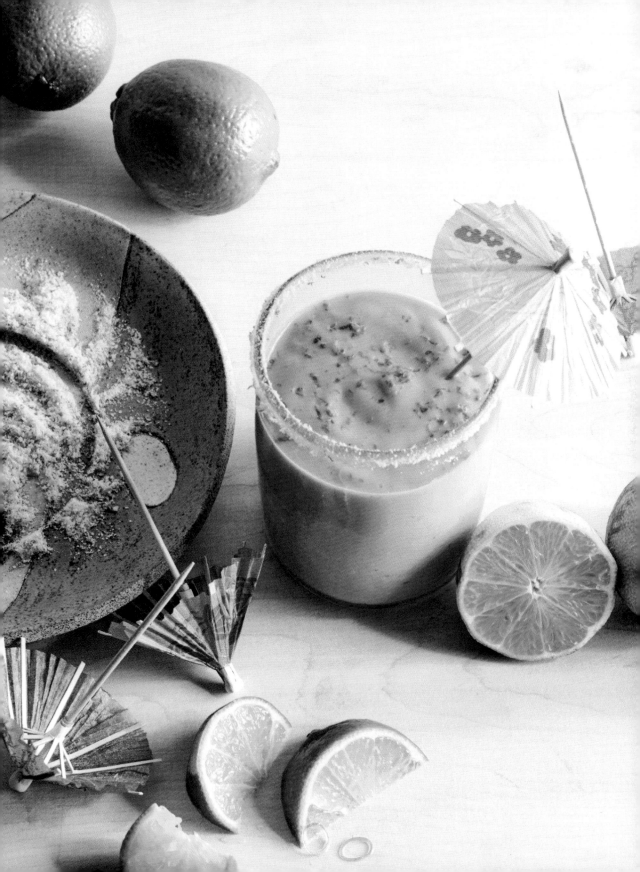

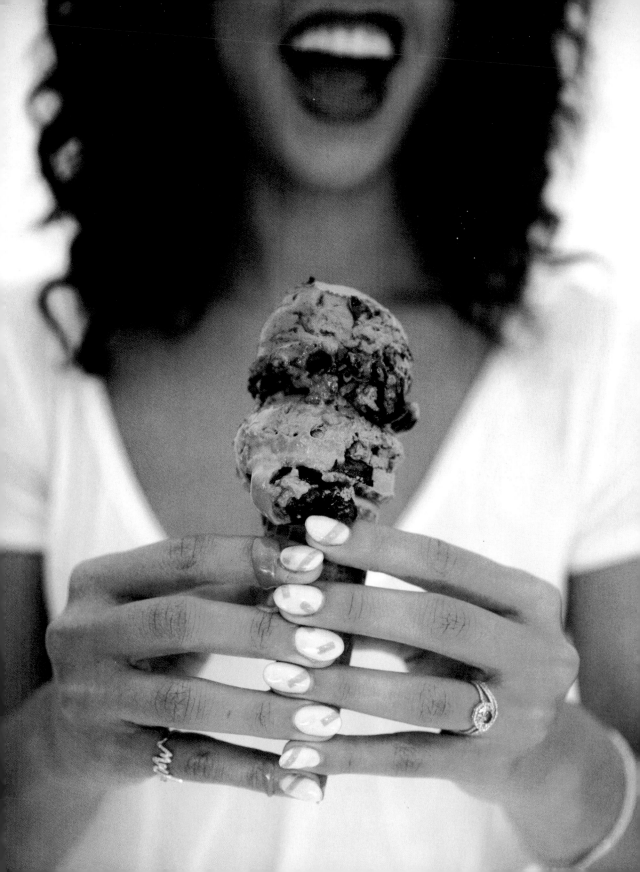

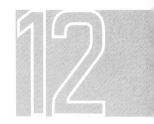

healthy
HEDONISM

DESSERTS AND SOMETHING EXTRA

SEX CHOCOLATES

do
what
feels
good

These chocolates can be made with your choice of two "love potion" bundles derived from adaptogenic herbs, like he shou wu for amping up desire and fertility, and Siberian ginseng for maximum energy and satisfaction. Or you can just make the chocolates without the herbs and you'll still get a nice dose of antioxidants from the dark chocolate and the cocoa powder. Either way, you'll forget about all of their health benefits the minute you take a bite—they are sinfully good. Beware, may cause sassiness.

Makes 9 to 15 truffles

1. Heat the coconut milk and herbs over low heat and let simmer, covered, for 15 minutes.

2. Remove the lid, add the chocolate to the pot, and stir constantly until the chocolate has melted.

3. Let cool until set; 2 to 3 hours in the refrigerator.

4. Using a tablespoon-size scoop, scoop truffles onto a plate.

5. Quickly roll between your hands to make perfectly round.

6. Toss the truffles in the cocoa powder to coat.

7. Serve immediately, or store in the refrigerator for 3 to 4 days. Let come to room temperature before serving.

YOU SAY COCOA, I SAY CACAO

Here's the drill on dark chocolate, cacao, and cocoa:[1] It all starts with cacao trees, which grow greenish-yellow football-shaped pods that are picked and split to reveal the beans. The raw beans are called cacao. Roasted beans become cocoa. Both can be turned into powders, bars, chips, nibs, drinks, or desserts. But cacao is the one with the amped-up health benefits, like antioxidants, or theobromine, which can improve your mood.

This doesn't mean that cocoa powder, made by grinding cocoa beans and removing most of the fat, is bad for you. Just remember that cocoa powder and Dutch-process cocoa powder (made by alkalizing the beans to remove some of the bitterness)[2] are not the same as hot co-coa mix, which has so much corn syrup that it doesn't even taste good.

When people say that chocolate is good for you, those health bene-fits are actually coming from cacao. So when choosing chocolate bars, aim for dark over milk, and look for those with a high percentage of cacao. For snacking or baking, choose cacao nibs, which deliver more antioxidants than chocolate chips do.

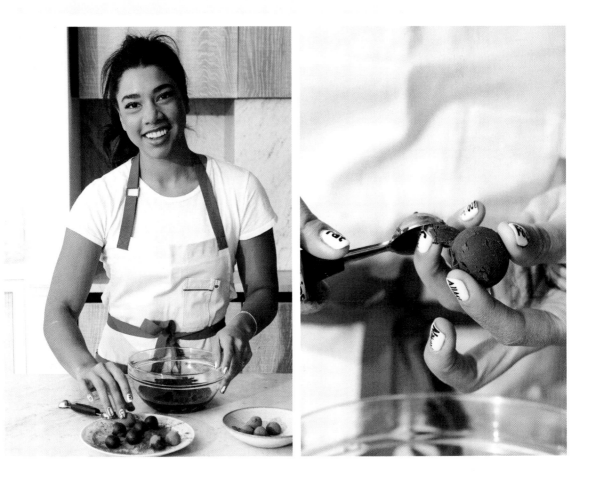

16-HOUR CANNABIS BUTTER

INGREDIENTS

½ pound unsalted grass-fed butter or coconut oil

1 cup water

½ ounce cannabis buds or flowers, finely ground (or ¾ ounce cannabis trim)

Up to 1 teaspoon sea salt (optional, see headnote)

If you're into cannabis edibles, this is the recipe for you. This infused butter can be used for cooking and baking or stirred into tea for an extra-relaxing evening. It's incredibly versatile. You can make it with coconut oil instead of butter, and you can add salt or not. I prefer unsalted pot butter for baking and salted for savory dishes. You can also use high-quality cannabis trim instead of buds if you'd like. Remember to use sparingly and responsibly for best effects. Eat responsibly and chill.

Makes ½ pound butter

1. Add the butter, salt, and water to a slow cooker and simmer on low, stirring occasionally, until the butter melts.*

2. When the butter has melted, add the cannabis buds.

3. Cover and cook on the lowest setting of your slow cooker for 16 hours.

4. Using a fine-mesh strainer lined with cheesecloth, strain the hot butter-water mixture into a refrigerator-safe glass container.

5. Store in the refrigerator overnight. When the butter is completely solid, it will separate from the water. Discard the water, saving the cannabis-infused butter.

6. Use in place of butter or oil in any of your favorite recipes—just remember: It's strong stuff!

*You can also do this over very low heat on the stovetop. Just simmer, covered, on low for 2 to 3 hours, then resume instructions at step 4.

do
what
feels
good

AVOCADO-CHOCOLATE MOUSSE

When I made this mousse for Action Bronson on his VICELAND show, *The Untitled Action Bronson Show*, he was totally freaked about the idea of avocados for dessert. Once he tasted it, though, he was blown away. This mousse is super light and fluffy, and if you use a good-quality cocoa powder, you will never taste a hint of avocado (not to hate on avocados—you know I love you—but I love chocolate more). If you don't want to use honey or agave to sweeten it, you can substitute 6 to 8 drops of liquid stevia. The key here is to whip the silky blend by hand to achieve the mousse-like consistency.

Serves 4

1. In a food processor fitted with an "S" blade, pulse the avocados until broken apart.

2. Add the honey, cocoa powder, milk, vanilla extract, and salt and blend until smooth.

3. Transfer to a bowl, and whip until a fluffy, mousse-like texture is achieved.

4. Fill four individual serving bowls with the mousse and top with the Coconut Whipped Cream and fresh berries.

INGREDIENTS

2 ripe avocados, pitted and peeled

$\frac{1}{4}$ cup mild honey or agave nectar

$\frac{1}{4}$ cup unsweetened natural (not Dutch-process) cocoa powder

2 tablespoons milk of your choice

1 teaspoon pure vanilla extract

$\frac{1}{8}$ teaspoon sea salt

Coconut Whipped Cream (page 229), for serving

Fresh berries, for serving

PUMPKIN PIE X COCONUT CREAM

INGREDIENTS

FOR THE CRUST

$\frac{1}{2}$ cup almonds

$\frac{1}{4}$ cup hulled pumpkin seeds

$\frac{1}{4}$ cup shredded unsweetened coconut flakes

$\frac{1}{2}$ cup diced pitted dates

1 teaspoon pure vanilla extract

$\frac{1}{2}$ teaspoon ground cinnamon

$\frac{1}{2}$ teaspoon sea salt

I've loved pumpkin for as long as I can remember. Pumpkin is the poster child for fall, and my birthday happens to land during peak pumpkin season, October 26. Coincidence? I think not. Fall pies are some of my favorites, and this vegan pumpkin pie will surprise you with its richness and decadence. Allow it to set overnight and be sure to get the Coconut Whipped Cream in order a half hour prior to serving. For the ultimate party pairing, serve up a slice with a side of Only Noni (page 217).

Serves 8 to 10

FIRST, MAKE THE CRUST

1. Place the almonds and pumpkin seeds in a food processor fitted with an "S" blade and pulse to a flour-like consistency.

2. Add the coconut and dates and continue to pulse until a sticky dough begins to form.

3. Add the remaining ingredients and pulse until a dough has formed that holds its shape when squeezed between two fingers.

4. Press the dough into the bottom of an 8-inch springform pan, and chill in the refrigerator until needed.

do
what
feels
good

NEXT, MAKE THE FILLING

1. Add the cherries to the milk and let sit for 20 minutes to soften.

2. Transfer to a high-speed blender or a food processor fitted with an "S" blade and blend until smooth.

3. Blend all the remaining ingredients except the pomegranate molasses and Coconut Whipped Cream into the cherry mixture until smooth. Taste, and adjust the sweetness by adding additional cherries or, if needed, a date.

4. Pour the filling into the prepared crust and let set in the refrigerator overnight.

5. Serve the pie, drizzled with the pomegranate molasses and topped with the Coconut Whipped Cream.

FOR THE FILLING

$\frac{1}{2}$ cup dried tart cherries

$\frac{1}{4}$ cup milk of your choice

$1\frac{3}{4}$ cups pure unsweetened pumpkin puree (canned okay)

$\frac{1}{4}$ cup melted coconut oil or grass-fed butter

1 teaspoon pure vanilla extract

$\frac{1}{4}$ teaspoon sea salt

$\frac{1}{4}$ cup pure maple syrup

$\frac{1}{3}$ teaspoon ground cinnamon

$\frac{1}{3}$ teaspoon ground ginger

$\frac{1}{3}$ teaspoon freshly grated nutmeg

$\frac{1}{3}$ teaspoon ground cloves

1 to 2 tablespoons pomegranate molasses, for serving

1 cup Coconut Whipped Cream (page 228), for serving

COCONUT WHIPPED CREAM

INGREDIENTS

1 can full-fat unsweetened coconut cream, refrigerated for 24 hours

1 vanilla bean, split

1 teaspoon pure maple syrup

If you are a whipped cream lover (and really, who isn't) and you're considering ditching dairy, I have to tell you: this stuff is so, so good. Yes, coconut whipped cream tastes "coconut-y," but that hint of nuttiness and sweetness just makes it even more delicious. You can put this whip on anything and everything—as a frosting for cakes, as a topping for pies and ice cream, or even as a crowning dollop for hot cocoa. I've also been known to just eat it by the spoonful (with or without almond butter).

Makes 2 cups

1. Chill a mixing bowl and a whisk in the freezer for 30 minutes.

2. Carefully open the can of coconut cream, scoop the solid white cream off the top, and place it in the chilled bowl. Save the coconut water for another use.

3. Scrape the seeds from the vanilla bean into the coconut cream, add the maple syrup, and whisk until it reaches the consistency of whipped cream.

4. Serve immediately.

do
what
feels
good

BLUEBERRY CHEESECAKE

This raw vegan cheesecake is the perfect dessert for summertime, when farmers' markets have all those cute little pint boxes brimming over with fresh, ripe blueberries. I love that this dessert isn't overly sweet—there's only ¼ cup of honey in the whole pie—and the orange and thyme add some depth and complexity. It's also a real stunner—you will be the toast of any soiree if you show up with this cake. And remember to take the compliment when you do!

Serves 8 to 10

1. Prepare the pie crust and refrigerate until needed.

2. Soak the cashews or macadamia nuts in water for 8 to 10 hours; overnight is perfect!

3. Drain the soaked nuts, and transfer to a food processor fitted with an "S" blade or a high-speed blender.

4. Add the lemon zest and juice, orange zest, thyme, blueberries, and coconut milk and process until blended.

5. Add the coconut oil, honey, salt, vanilla bean, and goji powder and process until completely smooth.

6. Taste, and add additional goji powder or blueberries for sweetness if needed.

7. Pour the filling into the prepared crust and transfer to the freezer for at least 2 hours, or the refrigerator for at least 6 hours, until set.

8. Unmold, and top with the ¼ cup fresh blueberries, thyme sprigs, and reserved lemon zest before serving.

INGREDIENTS

1 prepared raw pie crust, in an 8-inch springform pan (see Pumpkin Pie X Coconut Cream, page 226)

2 cups raw cashews or macadamia nuts

Finely grated zest and juice of 1 lemon (reserve some zest for garnish)

Finely grated zest of 1 orange

1 teaspoon fresh thyme leaves, plus thyme sprigs for garnish

¾ cup blueberries (fresh, or frozen and thawed), plus ¼ cup fresh berries for garnish

½ cup well-shaken canned, full-fat coconut milk

⅔ melted coconut oil or grass-fed butter

¼ cup mild raw honey

Pinch of sea salt

1 vanilla bean, seeds scraped

2 tablespoons goji powder (see Pink Beauty Butter, page 148)

MATCHA CHEESECAKE

1⅔ cups raw cashews or macadamia nuts

1 raw pie crust, patted into an 8-inch springform pan (see Pumpkin Pie X Coconut Cream, page 226)

¾ cup canned unsweetened coconut cream*

½ cup mild raw honey, agave nectar, or pure maple syrup

½ cup melted coconut oil or grass-fed butter

½ teaspoon pure vanilla extract

1½ tablespoons matcha powder, or more to taste

I've been on the matcha train for years now. I love the way it tastes, the way it makes me feel, and its amazing health benefits. In addition to my morning matcha latte routine (see page 57), I like to use matcha in my sweets. The earthiness of matcha provides such a nice balance in desserts. This raw matcha cheesecake is made with nuts and natural sweeteners for a dairy-free alternative to traditional cheesecake. The color is soooo dreamy that sometimes I find myself making it just for the gram. After all, they don't call me Matcha Stewart for nothing!

Serves 8 to 10

1. Soak the cashews or macadamia nuts in water for 2 to 8 hours.

2. Meanwhile, prepare the crust.

3. Drain the soaked nuts, and transfer to a food processor fitted with an "S" blade or a high-speed blender.

4. Add the coconut cream, honey, coconut oil, vanilla, and matcha powder and blend until very smooth.

5. Taste, and add more matcha powder, a tiny bit at a time, to your personal taste.

6. When the mixture is smooth and flavorful, pour it into the prepared crust.

7. Freeze for at least 2 hours, or refrigerate for 8 hours, until set, before slicing and serving.

8. Store leftovers in the refrigerator for up to 5 days.

*Carefully remove the solid coconut cream from the can with a spoon and save the thinner coconut water for another use.

do
what
feels
good

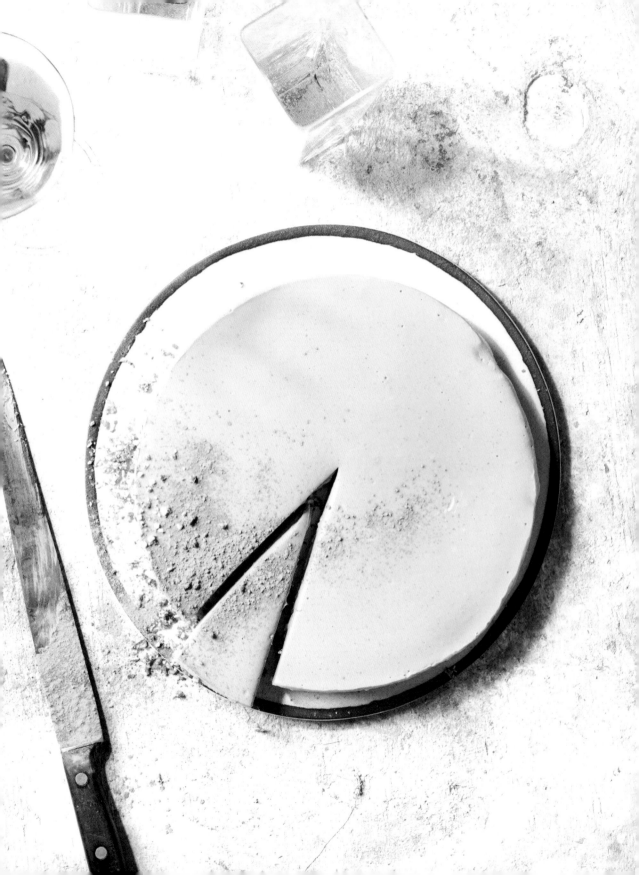

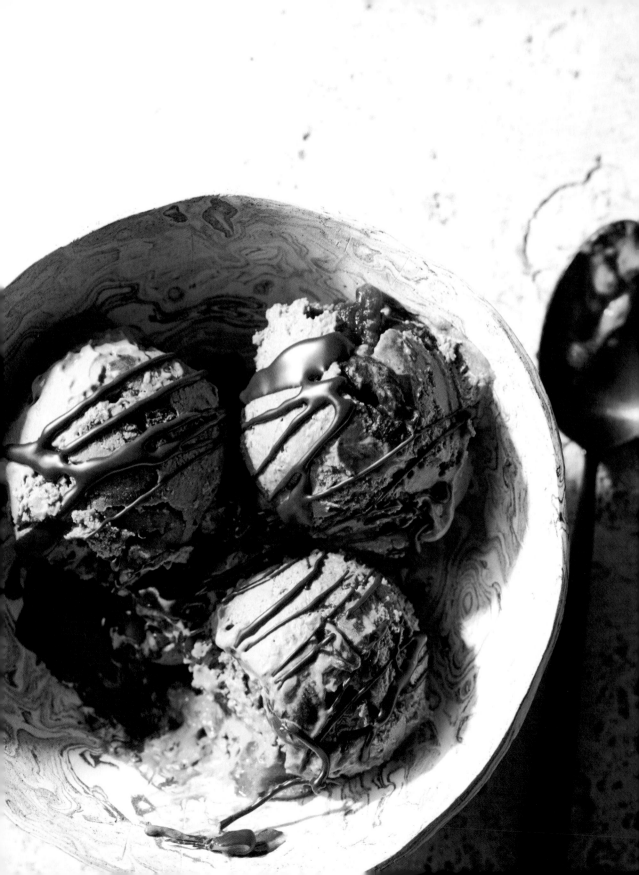

CHOCOLATE CHERRY CHUNK ICE DREAM

You would never believe this luscious frozen dessert is dairy-free. The secret ingredient? Avocado. With tart cherries, rich coconut cream, and bittersweet chocolate, you won't miss the cow's milk one bit. And it's so rich and satisfying that one scoop goes a long way!

Makes 1 pint

1. If it's not already in the freezer, chill the core of your ice cream machine until completely frozen (typically takes between 4 and 8 hours).

2. Add the coconut cream, cherry juice, monk fruit sweetener, and cocoa powder to a medium saucepan.

3. Whisk over medium heat until the monk fruit sweetener has completely dissolved, then add *half* of the chocolate chips.

4. Reduce the heat to low and continue to whisk until the chocolate has melted. Remove from the heat.

5. Transfer to a high-speed blender and add the vanilla and avocados. Blend until very smooth.

6. Pour into a bowl, cover, and refrigerate until very cold; at least 2 hours.

7. Stir in the remaining chocolate chips and the cherries, then spoon into the ice cream maker and churn until it reaches the consistency of soft-serve ice cream.

8. Serve immediately or freeze in a glass container to hard-serve consistency.

9. For leftovers, let come to scoopable temperature before serving.

*Can't find fresh sour cherries? Use dried sour cherries and reconstitute them in the cherry juice before using.

INGREDIENTS

1 (15-ounce) can unsweetened coconut cream

$\frac{1}{4}$ cup sour cherry juice

$\frac{3}{4}$ cup monk fruit sweetener

2 tablespoons unsweetened cocoa powder

6 ounces bittersweet chocolate chips

1 teaspoon pure vanilla extract

2 avocados, pitted and peeled

$\frac{1}{4}$ cup frozen, pitted sour cherries*

OLIVE OIL CAKE

1 unpeeled orange, quartered

Finely grated zest of 1 lemon

1 teaspoon fresh rosemary needles, plus sprigs for garnish

6 large eggs*

$\frac{2}{3}$ cup extra-virgin olive oil

$\frac{3}{4}$ cup mild honey or pure maple syrup

2 cups finely ground blanched almond flour

2 teaspoons baking powder

$\frac{1}{2}$ teaspoon sea salt

Thinly sliced oranges (raw or dehydrated), for garnish

Coconut Whipped Cream (page 228), for serving

When I was a kid, my dad and I shared the commonality that we didn't like traditional fancy cake consistency. (Obviously that excludes Betty Crocker box cake . . . I said *fancy*.) I love the texture of this rich, moist cake, which uses olive oil as the only fat. Lightly scented with lemon zest and rosemary, it is not very sweet yet it has a sophisticated enough flavor profile to be classified as a fancy cake. In fact, this cake is so fancy that it was the base for our wedding cake!

Serve 8 to 10

1. Preheat the oven to 325°F. Spray a 9-inch cake pan with olive oil and line with parchment paper. Set aside.

2. In a blender or a food processor fitted with an "S" blade, blend together the orange, lemon zest, rosemary, eggs, olive oil, and honey until smooth.

3. In a large bowl, whisk together the almond flour, baking powder, and sea salt.

4. Pour the orange mixture into the almond mixture and mix until just combined.

5. Transfer to the prepared pan and bake for 30 to 35 minutes, or until the edges of the cake pull away from the sides of the pan and a sharp knife inserted into the center comes out clean.

6. Cool to room temperature, and serve topped with the thinly sliced oranges, rosemary sprigs, and Coconut Whipped Cream.

*If you'd like a denser cake, use only 4 eggs.

do
what
feels
good

WORLD'S EASIEST ALMOND COOKIES

Major crowd-pleaser. These little cookies were everyone's favorite at our photo shoot—they disappeared from the set minutes after we'd finished shooting them! They're light and crispy and just sweet enough. They're the perfect treat to bring to a party or picnic, as they hold up well for traveling.

Makes 12 to 16 cookies

1. Preheat the oven to 350°F. Line 2 cookie sheets with parchment paper and set aside.

2. Make the rosemary simple syrup: Simmer ½ cup of maple syrup with 1 tablespoon fresh rosemary over low heat for 10 to 15 minutes. Strain and let it cool.

3. Whisk the almond flour and baking powder together in a large bowl.

4. Add the cooled syrup, orange zest, and vanilla extract and stir until a sticky dough has formed.

5. Drop rounded tablespoons of the dough onto the prepared cookie sheets, spacing them 1 to 2 inches apart.

6. Sprinkle the top of each cookie with the sliced almonds.

7. Bake for 11 to 12 minutes. Cool before serving.

INGREDIENTS

$\frac{1}{3}$ cup rosemary simple syrup (see step 2)

2 cups finely ground blanched almond flour

$\frac{1}{2}$ teaspoon baking powder

Finely grated zest of 1 orange

2 teaspoons pure vanilla extract

$\frac{1}{2}$ cup sliced almonds

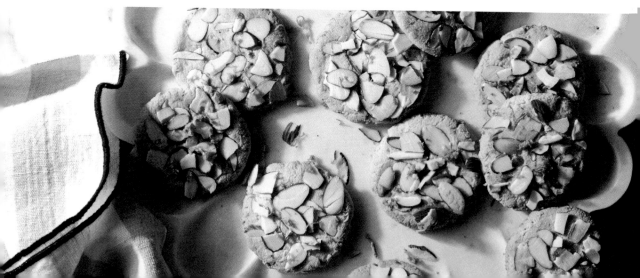

CHOCOLATE-ALMOND BUTTER CUPS

INGREDIENTS

$\frac{1}{2}$ cup smooth almond butter

1 tablespoon pure maple syrup

$\frac{1}{2}$ teaspoon ground cinnamon

$\frac{1}{4}$ teaspoon sea salt

1 tablespoon coconut flour

2 cups bittersweet chocolate chips (or chopped bittersweet chocolate)

$1\frac{1}{2}$ tablespoons coconut oil

Flaky sea salt, such as Maldon, for garnish

Almond butter is a staple in my pantry and in my diet. It's high in protein, easy to tote around, and so, so good. Here, it serves as the primary ingredient in a perfect little bite-size dessert that is a much healthier take on our favorite name-brand treats.

Makes 24 cups

1. Line a mini muffin pan with paper liners and set aside.

2. In a bowl, whisk together the almond butter, maple syrup, cinnamon, sea salt, and coconut flour until well combined; a smooth, thickish paste should form. Cover and chill in the refrigerator or freezer until thickened; 10 to 15 minutes.

3. Remove from the freezer and roll into a log. Break into 24 equal pieces and mold each piece into a flat disk slightly smaller than the cups in the muffin pan. Set aside.

4. Melt together the chocolate chips and coconut oil over a double boiler or in a microwave in 10-second increments, stirring until smooth.

5. Drop a teaspoon of melted chocolate into each of the prepared cups, and shake/tap the pan to create a smooth, even layer.

6. Place the disks of filling on top of the chocolate, and top with the remaining chocolate. Tap to eliminate air bubbles.

7. Sprinkle with the flaky salt and freeze until set. Let come to room temperature before serving.

do
what
feels
good

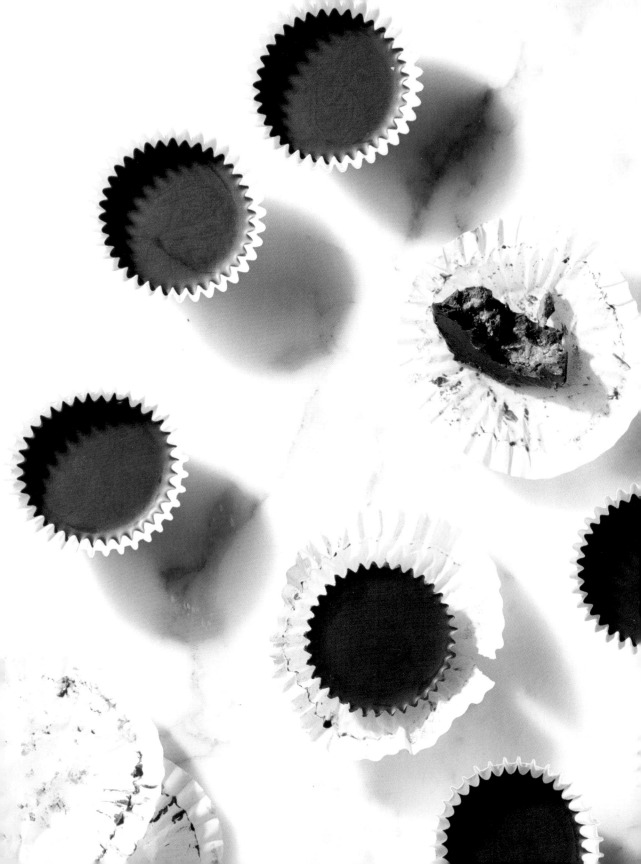

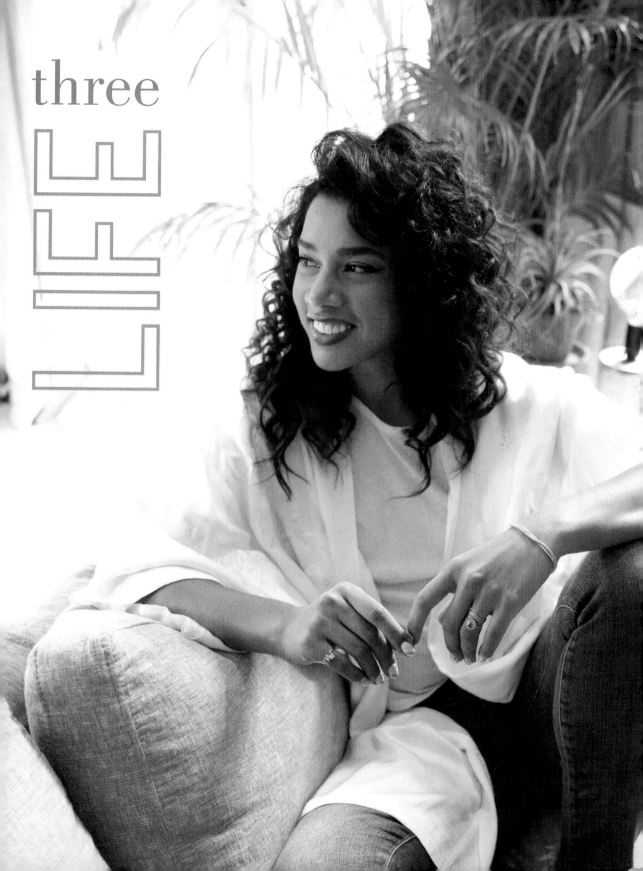

three

LIFE

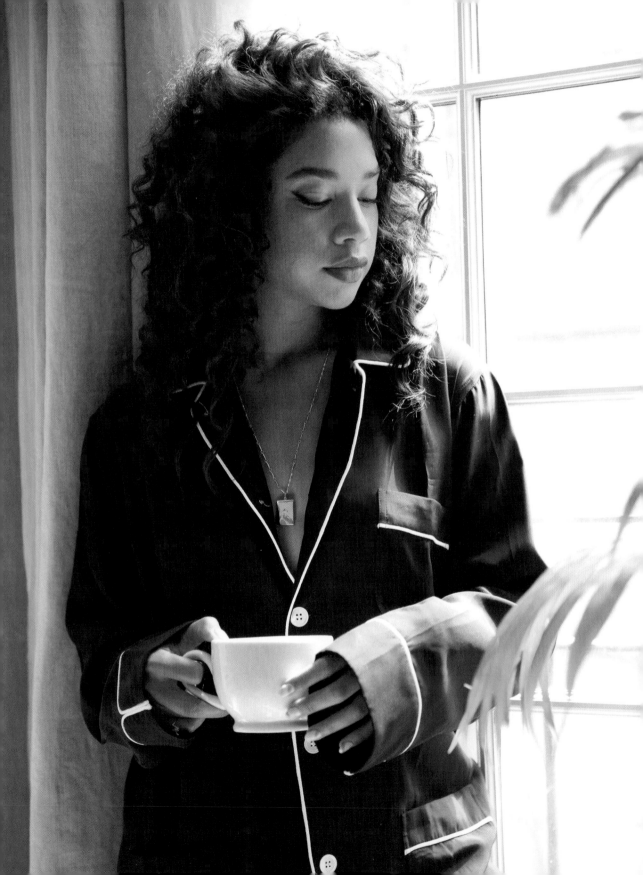

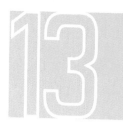

do it and do it and do it AGAIN

ROUTINES ARE KEY

Every single day, when I wake up in the morning, I pour myself a big glass of room-temperature water and gulp it down. (Everyone says that you should sip, but I gulp.) That glass of water in the morning is as routine for me as washing my face. I drink it whether or not I feel thirsty in the moment because I know it will help to wake up my body (and my digestion) after a night's rest. I drink room-temperature water because cold water actually slows down your digestion and you always want to keep that train moving at full speed.

For me, starting the day with a glass of water is a reminder to be conscious about my actions, and it impacts me for the rest of the day. Making one strong move in the a.m. leads me to the next move, and so on. And as long as I'm in tune with my body in the morning, my day can settle into the rhythm that lets me feel my best all day long.

Some of you might be thinking, "But I like to mix things up, I don't want a 'routine'!" I feel you. I don't have a typical job, so my schedule is a little different every day. But my routines—water first thing when I wake up, tea or tonic, taking my daily supplements, washing my face and moisturizing my skin, getting my heart rate up or stretching my body: those are my consistencies. My routines are built around the idea that, no matter how busy I get, basic self-care is an essential part of my day.

Those times when I'm in sync with myself help me feel my best so I can do my best. I can run my business and be ready to respond as I need to. I can show up, with all of my energy, to whatever I'm doing: working, working out, hanging out with friends and family, spending time with my husband. I can also bring that enthusiasm to my self-care.

I'm a very results-driven person, so I'm constantly assessing and reassessing and honing my routines. What I've discovered over the past few years is that the only way for me to know if a habit is actually going to help me get results that are lasting and worthwhile is to do it again and again. If I add or modify a routine in some way, I do that same thing repeatedly to see what kind of results it's giving me. This is where being consistently aware of the way I feel comes in handy. I pay attention to how I feel before, during, and after I institute that change. That's the only way I can really know if something's working.

I love a routine because it takes the pressure off. Once I've figured out what works for me, I can just do it every day without thinking about it. And that frees up my energy to focus on all the other things I want to do.

WAIT, WHAT?

Early in my health journey, Tracy Piper asked me to try something new that she thought would be really beneficial for my digestion: First, she wanted me to drink water as soon as I woke up each day (check). But she also wanted me to abstain from drinking water thirty minutes before a meal and wait forty-five minutes after I had eaten to drink again.

Excuse me?

She was serious. I was no longer supposed to eat and drink at the same time.

I would drink all of my water throughout the day at times when I wasn't having food. That made me nervous. It would be easy enough to drink more water in the morning, I thought, but no more water with my lunch? How was that going to work? What if I ate throughout the day? How would I handle it?

At this point in my life, I'm a happy guinea pig. I'll try anything. But at the beginning of my health journey, I was warier. I wasn't as ready to make changes—even though I was sure something needed to change. It just made no sense to me! But I really trusted Tracy, and I knew she had my best interests at heart (just like I do for you). So I let what she was saying sink in. I knew I would like it if I saw that it was giving me results.

It was a little weird at the beginning to push away the glass of water that is inevitably poured for you at mealtimes, but I did it. I would make sure to drink plenty of water well before lunch. Avoid water while I ate. And then forty-five minutes later, I would have my water. I did the same in the evenings.

And wow! Drinking water throughout the day, at the right times, had a remarkable effect on my awareness of when I am truly hungry and when I am in need of hydration. Having that time to focus on food,

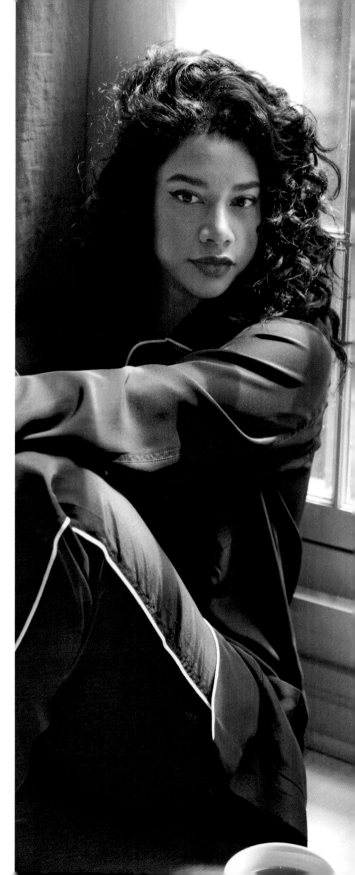

without the distraction of adding liquid to the mix, let me experience how it felt to be full and nourished, not just full of liquid. Then forty or fifty minutes later, I would be truly thirsty, and I could really enjoy that glass of water. And I was drinking a lot more water, too, which kept my belly full and kept my digestion regular.

And, BTW, it was weirdly empowering to take charge of my routine in this way. Becoming conscious about my hydration helped me on so many levels. Being able to actively shift this very small thing in order to create change was satisfying and also, on some level, a relief. Looking back, I can see that changing my whole life so that I could become healthier took years of trial and error. Training myself to drink water at

the right times was a cakewalk by comparison.

I still believe that this routine was part of what cracked the self-care code for me. At first, I had to concentrate. I had to remind myself. It took a little while to get used to. Now I can't imagine not doing this. I have fewer headaches when I'm hydrated, and more energy. I can tell I love this routine because I keep it up now, without even really thinking about it, eight years later. And no matter how my eating habits might change, as I experiment with different ways of nourishing myself with food, I stick with my water routine.

It's my basic. It's my white T-shirt. It's my jeans. It's my favorite boots that I want to wear every day.

> I still believe that this routine was part of what cracked the self-care code for me.

MY HYDRATION ROUTINE

I hear a lot of people talk about how hard it is to make time for fitness or to prep healthy food for themselves. I hear you, man. It is really challenging to make time for those things. But drinking water is pretty easy. Water is something you need to stay alive, and you're (hopefully) drinking it regularly anyways, so why not see if shifting your intake impacts how you feel? If it doesn't, no biggie. But if you do feel a difference, or if you learn something about your body and about yourself, win-win, right?

Everyone says it takes twenty-one days to implement a habit. But honestly, this one only takes a couple of days. Drinking water more consciously was my first step into a new routine that became the foundation of my healthier lifestyle, which is why I offer the basics of my water routine to you now:

- I drink water all day, except around meals.
- I drink a glass of room-temperature water first thing in the morning.
- I always leave water by my bedside.
- I aim for two liters a day—one before lunch and one in the afternoon/evening.
- I don't drink while I eat. Thirty minutes before a meal, I stop drinking water. Forty-five minutes after a meal, I have a glass of water.
- I keep it classic: no ice, no carbonation, room temperature.
- I like drinking out of a glass jar.
- I drink water—a lot of water—while working out.
- I always have a big bottle with me, wherever I go.
- When I travel, before I get to my hotel, I stop at a market and buy a few bottles of water to keep in my room.

THIRSTY FOR IT

When your brain senses an impending water emergency, it lets you know. Your mouth gets dry, and you may start to lick your lips. This is a sign to put down the Chapstick and reach for a glass. Thirst is your body basically sending emergency flares like, HEY ARE YOU THERE? WTF? For the love of Beyoncé, just drink something already!!

Maybe I still haven't swayed you. You're used to drinking enough water to avoid dying, but you're still not planning to drag a bottle of water around to make sure you get adequate hydration. Well, listen, let me tell you a little bit about why water is so important, even if you're tempted to flip to another chapter right now (possibly "cocktails"). Because, personally, when I know the "why" behind something, I'm more likely to make a change to my routines that sticks. So let's take a quick minute to talk about why you need to drink more water, starting right now.

More than half of your body—in fact, 60 percent—is water, and if you want to thrive, it needs to stay that way. Water is the most essential nutrient (yes, water is considered a nutrient) for your survival. Even though when you're hungry, you can feel like you're going to die if you don't eat something within a few minutes, the body can actually survive for about three weeks without food (not that any of us have any interest in testing this out) because it can live off reserved fat stores for a while. But you can only last a few *days* without water. And the side effects of dehydration, even in the short term—messed-up concentration and memory, headaches, feeling tired and angry, having sore muscles—are no joke.

I know, I know, it might seem obvious or even kind of annoying to devote this much space in a book to *water*. How many interviews have you read with celebrities who look amazing and swear their only beauty "secret" is drinking water? I get it. I roll my eyes, too. But the thing is, hydra-tion is one of those things that is so easy to overlook. We pay a lot of attention to the food we eat with a knife and fork, but we don't always pay as much attention to what we're sipping on. Oftentimes those things are jam-packed with sugar, caffeine, or booze when what we really need is water. And yes, your body can use the water in teas, broths, and fresh fruits and vegetables, but the best source is pure water. I know people who could list every vegetable they've eaten all day long, but if you asked them the last time they had a sip of water, they'd be like "Ummm, this morning after yoga?" For all of their nutritional virtuousness, they're missing out on the most important one. So remember: Sometimes it's the easiest thing that we don't pay attention to that can make the biggest difference.

ALL ROUTINES HAVE RESULTS

Feeling good starts with what you do every day. What do you do that makes you feel like you? What do you do that gets in the way of feeling good? We all need to do more of what works, less of what doesn't.

Take a minute and think about your routines and how they set you up for success—or not. What habits or daily choices are a part of your routines? Which parts of those routines are adding up to strength, to well-being, to feeling good, and which are making you feel worse? Are your routines giving you the results you want? If not, what could you substitute that might support your goals?

We all have routines, even if we're not consciously aware of them. But it's important to become aware because how you feel right now is largely the result of your routines. If you're not super psyched about the results—if you're not feeling good most of the time—then I beg you: Change the routines! Why waste your time and your energy on shitty routines that work against you?

I'm not just talking about super-unhealthy routines. You might have a cereal-for-dinner routine or a strict no-breakfast routine. And what about those seemingly beneficial routines? If you're bored by eating the same salad every day, injured from exercising too much, or tired from getting up at the crack of dawn to be more productive, your "healthy" routine isn't working for you either. And it sure as hell isn't making you feel good.

YA GOTTA START SOMEWHERE

In order to get healthy, over time, I had to take a look at my schedule, my goals, my attitudes and beliefs, and my less-than-good habits. I had to shift my priorities. I had to find teachers. I had to be willing to ask questions—and to listen to the answers. And then I had to get real. Honestly, it was really hard.

That's why the easiest routine changes were such major touchstones for me. I had to reorganize my life around better routines, ones that would benefit me instead of break me down. But since changing too many things at once can be confusing and intimidating, it helped me to focus on the simplest specifics. Like making my tonics. Like swapping dairy for nut milks. Like eating more vegetables. I could do these things, and the results kept me inspired on my journey to make deeper, lasting changes.

Think about change like a muscle in your body. The more you exercise it, the more elastic it gets and the more flexible you are when it comes to trying new things. So, at the beginning, the idea of trying something new might make your heart beat a little faster. You might want to say no just because change is uncomfortable. Trying on a new routine isn't easy, and you might be tempted to return to your old ways.

Start with one thing. Make a small change, be consistent with it, and see how it affects you. The more aware you become of your daily choices and default behavior patterns, the better you can fine-tune a routine that supports your goals and delivers results.

LET THE RHYTHM MOVE YOU

I like to think of routine like rhythm. It's a consistent pattern, an energy, a way of moving. It hits you at an unconscious level. You wouldn't listen to a song with an annoying beat all day long—so why would you keep up a routine that you don't vibe with?

Ask yourself:

- What are four things you do consistently every day? (This could be eating habits, communication habits, sleep habits, movement habits, etc.)
- How do those things make you feel?

- Is there a habit you can add that would support your goals? Start with one small thing.
- How does this make you feel? Does it help you reach your goals?

I encourage you to keep a journal or a notebook to jot down how you feel as you tweak your routine. Maybe instead of your 4:00 latte order you decide to make yourself some tea and take a brisk 10-minute walk. Or maybe you decide to go to bed 30 minutes earlier each night. Whatever it is, keep track of how small changes make you feel. And build a new rhythm that moves you in the direction of feeling good.

CURATING A CUSTOM ROUTINE

To curate your best routine, you don't need to hire a drill sergeant to stand over your bed and blow a whistle at 4 a.m. sharp, instructing you to do push-ups while sipping adaptogenic tonics. I'm not into routines that dominate my life and stress me out. I didn't want to go through my day thinking about what I'm "supposed to be" doing.

It's also important to remember that your routine should evolve with your needs. I try to continually tweak my rou-

tine for the most benefit. It's an ongoing project, a work in progress, because it is based on listening to my body instead of following a set of rules. I eat mostly whole foods, the foods that make me feel good. I avoid dairy and gluten and processed sugars because I've seen that they affect me in negative ways. I try to move my body in a way that feels good most days of the week. And I have my water routine. That's about it.

do
what
feels
good

I can't tell you what your routine should be because I'm not you, and I don't know what your body needs to feel good. So instead of mapping out a routine for you, I want to offer some guidelines that might be helpful as you think about curating a routine that works for YOU.

• prioritize health. You've got to know what you want in order to create a pathway toward it. You've got to know where you want to go in order to begin your journey. As I learned the hard way, if your goal is to feel good (or even just feel better), health must be a priority.

• talk to yourself. How you feel is going to shift every day, and it's important to monitor that, to check in with yourself. As you begin to learn more about your needs, you can anticipate them and respond to changes as they arise.

• make space. What do you make room for? What do you make time for? A good routine always includes time for fitness, time for healthy eating, time for getting enough sleep—as well as all the other stuff we do.

• be open to learning something new. Find teachers. Read books. Ask questions. Indulge your curiosity. See who has the information that you need and ask them to tell you more.

• find the things you like. You can only do this by being a guinea pig and trying new things. If that isn't in your comfort zone, start small. Try one new thing. See how it makes you feel. Remember that it's *your* routine—you can change it if isn't working for you.

• take your pulse, and if you need to, take a pause. It's important to check your reactions. Not every supplement will work for you. Some types of exercise won't feel right. Give yourself what's good for you—which is not necessarily what's good for others.

• organize your home around your routines. If you want a glass of water in the morning, keep a pitcher near your bed. If you can only think clearly in a calm and organized home, cleanse your space regularly so you can fully chill and be more attuned to your needs.

• anticipate your meals. Go grocery shopping on a relaxing Sunday and spend some time either preparing your meals for the week or writing out what you'll be making each day.

• map out a realistic plan. Plan activities you can access with ease. Hiking is a wonderful way of working out, but not if it takes two hours to drive to a mountain. Find a class that works with your schedule. Hit the gym before the office, or pack lunch to eat at your desk and use lunchtime for gym time. Bike to brunch instead of taking public transportation. Walk instead of driving. Planning for accessible fitness makes it more likely that you'll engage in fitness.

• put yourself first. Routines are a part of self-care. They are about helping yourself, healing yourself, giving yourself what you need to feel good now, tomorrow, and the days after that.

CREATING A DEN OF PERSONAL ZEN

When I come home after another crazy day, I like to settle down on the couch with a cup of tea. It helps me relax and allows me to mark a space between work time and my time. I like to sit in my living room and catch up with my man without a phone in hand. If I happen to have an evening to myself, I am most definitely taking my tea to the bathroom and looking to see what mask I may want to try or potentially drawing myself a bath (more on that soon). Whatever I decide to do, whether it's stretching or cooking or just chilling on the couch, I try to take a moment for myself to just unwind from the day.

My home is the foundation of how I feel. When my personal space is organized, I feel like I've got my shit together.

> I believe in cleansing for the home just like I believe in it for my body. It's a cleansing for your soul.

When I feel like I've got my shit together, it's easier to keep my shit together. Creating a den of Zen at home is part of why I can be creative and organized about my work. It's why I can show up on time to meetings (most of the time). It's why I can make it to my fitness classes with my gym bag full of everything I'll need.

I know some people who lean toward living with clutter, who like having lots of things around. If that's your thing, then having a lot of stuff in your space will energize you and make it easier to adjust your routines as you need to. We all feel Zen in different spaces! My mom loves to have lots of things around her. She has every single umbrella that's ever existed and that any one of her children has ever owned. Her collection of umbrellas is so deep it's crazy. (But if you borrow one, she will notice!)

When I have too many things around, I start feeling uncomfortable. It makes me feel heavy, like I am carrying around stuff that I need to let go of. If I'm in a mode where I want to create change, changing what I see around me is often the best motivation for me.

Clearing my space is part of my routine. I believe in cleansing for home just like I believe in it for my body. It's a kind of cleansing for your soul. We get so full of old feelings, old attachments, old things—they can make us feel bloated emotionally. And I don't want to feel bloated physically or psychically. For me, extra stuff feels like unnecessary emotional weight. Just like I do with routines that don't help me, I want to cut the cords that are attaching me to the physical things that don't serve me. I want to get rid of what I don't need in order to make room for what I really want.

I think it's important to clear out the physical baggage when you're trying to make healthy changes, and your space sets the tone for your mood. It's a lot easier to stick to my conscious routines when I'm not distracted by chaos. If you're working on adding positive routines to your life, creating a home that supports how you want to feel can help.

SAY NO TO SAY YES

It's easy to say you're going to make a change—like eating more vegetables, or drinking more water, or moving your body more often, or getting more sleep—but it's really hard to be consistent with those changes when life gets in the way.

In order to do that, you have to be willing to make YOURSELF a priority. It's not easy to get out of a bad routine you're stuck in (which we actually call a rut). It takes time and energy, and if your energy is constantly being redirected by other people's needs, you can't spend it where you need to: on yourself.

I learned the value of choosing how I spend my time when I first started DJing. Someone would reach out with a request I wasn't interested in, and even when I knew that I should say no, even when I wanted to say no, I would say yes. In the back of my head, I'd know I had something else planned, but I couldn't say the word "no."

"Can you do it?"

"Yes!"

Every time.

"Can you do it?"

Say no, say no, I'd be thinking.

"Sure, I'll be there."

Yes. Yes. Yes.

I didn't know my own value or my own self-worth, and I let a lot of people take advantage of me. I gave away my time when I didn't want to, because, I thought, I'm new at this and I need to pay my dues. Which I did need to do, to an extent, but saying yes to so many other people left me less and less time to do what I needed for myself.

So I did what we often have to do when we find ourselves slipping into a routine that isn't working. I took a good look at what was going on, what I needed out of the situation, and what I could do to get myself there. And now I'm finding the older I get, the more my responsibilities extend to other people, and finding time for self-care is even more critical.

Ask yourself: What does it mean to say yes to *you*?

To me it means that my fitness is a priority and so is my nutrition and so is my rest, and that isn't because I'm selfish.

It's because I love myself and also because I love all the people in my life, from my husband to my parents to my besties. If I were to give up my fitness in order to cram something else into my schedule, how does that help me be my best and do my best in my interactions with those people? It wouldn't. Working out is such a great stress reliever and always elevates my mood—skipping too many sessions in a row makes me feel edgy.

All around me, I see women who are overextending themselves and giving away their time for free. And as we grow up and take on more and more responsibility, the list of what we'll be doing for others will get longer and longer. Self-care every day, people, is the only way through. Your well-being translates into the well-being of others. Paradoxically, that can sometimes look like you are saying NO.

But really, you are saying YES to yourself, to your health.

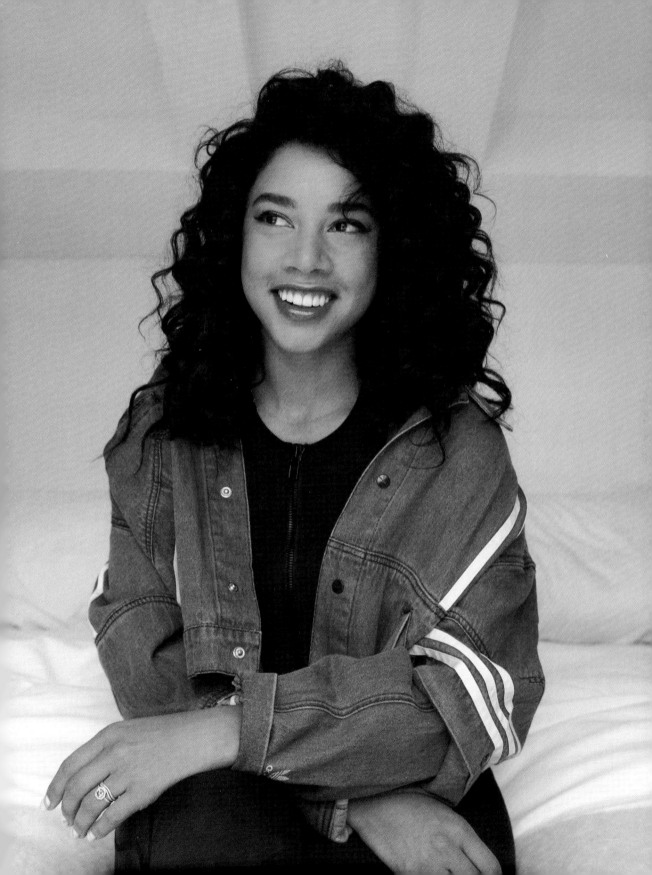

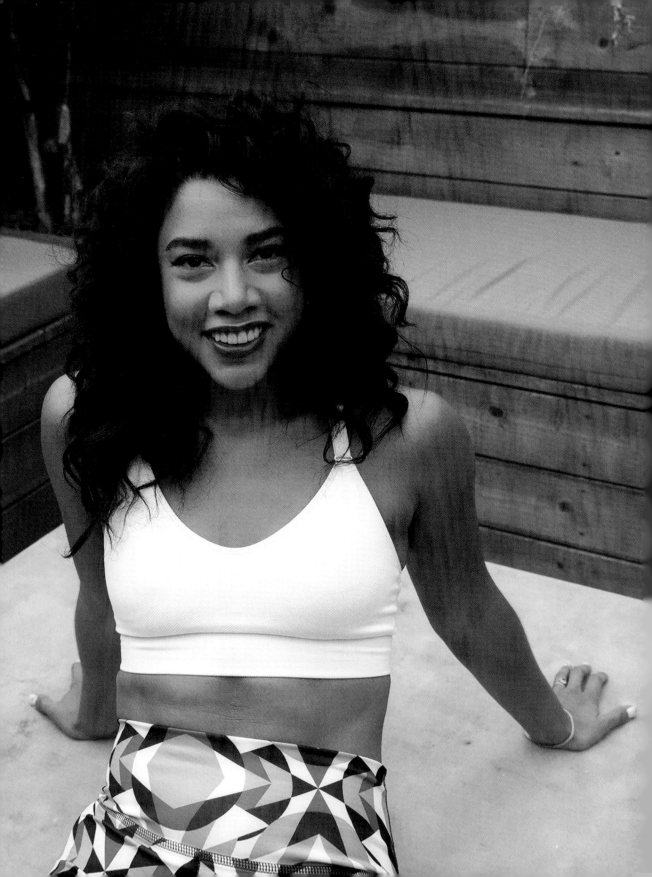

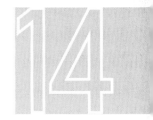

#FITFAM

GET UP AND MOVE (BUT REST DAYS, TOO)

A few years ago, Brendan and I went to Colorado for a little vacation. As a city girl who is always surrounded by the concrete jungle, I'll take any opportunity I can to get out into nature. We planned an eleven-mile hike to a beautiful lake. We packed lunches. It was gorgeous, all blue skies and sunshine, and we couldn't have been happier. Mile one, mile two, we were full of energy and basking in the landscape. And then we got lost.

We had already walked a mile in the wrong direction when we finally realized that we were no longer on the path. As we started backtracking, the weather changed and the sun disappeared. By the time we found the lake we were freezing. But we were there, so we just ate our lunches and had a look around. It was beautiful. It was breathtaking. We had hiked 3,000 feet in altitude, and we had made it, together.

When we finally got back to the place where we were staying, we kept talking about how incredible the whole experience was, including the wrong turns. And it was. It was actually a very difficult hike and I've never been so sore in my life, but we had our time together and we got to experience this amazing setting and the satisfaction of exploring the unknown and finding our way back home.

I love moments like this. I love when life and fitness merge together into one cohesive experience. For me, moving and challenging my body is a cornerstone of feeling good. Fitness isn't just something I want to do with a trainer so I can get an efficient workout. It isn't just something I want to do with a timer so I can keep track of my thirty-minute sprints. It's something I want to do so I can feel more like myself and have a better experience in my day and in my life.

That's what I want from my fitness routine. I always want my fitness to feel like a part of who I am and how I want to grow, whether I'm in a class or in my living room or lost on a mountaintop with the man I love. It took time to get there, though. I didn't always understand that fitness was about feeling fully like myself. When I was younger, I thought it was about transforming into someone else.

AIN'T NOBODY IN HERE STOPPING YOU

My earliest exposure to fitness came in the form of ballet classes, which I began at the tender age of four. It was a formative experience for me—physically and emotionally. It was pretty much just the basics at that age, but as I grew older I became hyper-aware of the body standards of the dance world. Every young girl was trying to be skinnier than the girl next to her. It was terrifying.

I have always loved to dance, and I still love the feeling of moving my body to the rhythm of music. But at some point, I started to fall out of love with ballet and the way it made me feel. I never felt I looked the part, and more important I did not feel the part. My legs were not as thin as those of the other girls, and I had a booty. I felt like I was being called out a lot in class, and despite how hard I was trying, I just wasn't getting my leg up high enough or I wasn't landing my turns perfectly. By age fifteen, it was clear that I wasn't going to be a professional ballerina. When I told my mom that I wanted to leave my ballet school, she said she was proud of me for standing up for myself in an environment that was damaging my health and my self-esteem. So I quit.

I still wanted to be physically active, though. What's a former ballerina to do? I was still drawn to challenging and competitive athletics, but with one key difference: I wanted to be part of a team. In high school, I joined the dance team, tennis team, and track team. I loved how collaborative team sports were. I liked engaging with the other players. I liked how everybody was able to have their own strengths and abilities, and that each of those strengths made us collectively stronger. That environment gave me the opportunity to develop more than just muscles. It also allowed me, as a young woman, to develop confidence. Leadership skills. Listening skills.

After college, I discovered the joys of other kinds of fitness that I never imagined doing before, like boxing. When I first started boxing, I was kind of timid. I wasn't hitting with all my strength, and it took me a while to understand my power. I realized, after a while, that it actually feels kind of amazing to hit something in a safe space. Boxing challenged my body and helped me understand my physical power. It cleared my head and it was so good for my soul. But it took time, and to get to all of these awesome feelings, I had to get over the weird, awkward feelings of being a fish out of water.

Anytime you start a new fitness routine, you'll see people all around you who are more expert than you. They know the moves, the timing; they have the strength to execute. I'll admit that sometimes my early ballet memories and habits emerge in this type of setting: that thing of comparing myself to other people, even though I know I don't need to. In a group class or in any situation, if I catch myself looking around the room and having negative feelings about myself based on someone else's abilities, I try to remember that in life there will always be people who are stronger or smarter or cooler or fitter—and that's fine. It's great, actually. Someone else's strength doesn't mean I can't become stronger. I want to surround

> I want to surround myself with people who are inspiring, and to let their awesomeness inspire motivation, not envy.

myself with people who are inspiring, and to let their awesomeness inspire motivation, not envy. Just like with team sports, a strong player makes the rest of us stronger. So give it your best energy no matter where you think you fall on the "Who's the best in here?" list. It doesn't matter. What matters is how much effort you put in. If you really go for it, you might even wind up inspiring someone else to try harder.

Because the energy of the pack—even if we are all strangers—is infectious. Whether you're just starting out or you're a fitness pro, everyone sweating in a room together has at least one thing in common: We are all there to do something that will allow us to leave class feeling a little bit better than when we walked in the door. We all want to feel good.

WHY I WORK OUT

So many people walk around all day long feeling like crap—I know because I used to be one of those people. Now I know that the quickest and most reliable antidote to a crappy day, for me, is moving my body. Every time I exercise, I can feel it working for me.

When I talk about "exercise," I'm referring to being active, and for every single person, that will look different in real life. Some people run Iron Men and some do Zumba. Some might lift 2-pound dumbbells while others are Crossfit champs. Some people are obsessed with high-intensity cardio, and some want to chill out with some gentle yoga. Any way you move your body is the right way if it's working for you.

For me, being physically active is about

constantly challenging myself and pushing my limits. Yes, that type of challenge affects the shape of my body, and I won't lie—visual results are motivating for me. Someone once told me that what you eat affects your weight, but how you move affects your shape. In my experience, this is 100 percent truth. My weight has more or less always remained the same, but my body has gone through several different shapes and muscle tonality over the years, all based on the fitness I was engaging with at the time.

But fitness is also something I choose so I can feel powerful and alive in my body. These experiences remind me that my body is a gift, that it is mine to do with as I please, that the mental and the physical are one and the same. What I know to be true is that fitness affects my whole life. It makes me feel tougher and stronger. It gives me energy and mental clarity. It helps me manage my mood, and I've found that different types of workouts have different effects on my mood. Running can be meditative. Boxing gives me focus and helps me release aggression. Different kinds of yoga can either wake me up and put me on a higher vibe or relax me and help me wind down.

There's so much research that supports what I know to be true experientially: fitness is good for your brain and your whole body. Cardio improves memory, cognition, and awareness.[1] Fitness helps with stress and anxiety. Doctors prescribe exercise if you want to prevent heart attacks, cancer, diabetes, depression, and more.[2] It's like taking blood pressure medication without a pill. Antidepressants without a pill. Heart medication without a pill. If you've got a chronic condition, it may be a drug-free care alternative and can also be used along with medication to help relieve side

effects of the drugs you may be taking.[3] And if you're looking for a sweet night's sleep, fitness is good for that, too.

I just celebrated my thirtieth birthday and I'm starting to wonder how I'll feel when the cake has forty candles in it. Lucky for me, my fitness routine is the best way for me to keep building bone now until I'm thirty-five, and to keep building muscle afterward. The truth is that people who don't exercise lose muscle mass every decade, while people who work out regularly can keep building muscle well into old age.

Plus, fitness literally makes your cells younger. All of our DNA has protective tips called telomeres that signal your biologic age. People who work out regularly have longer telomeres, which means more cellular protection, and a healthier prognosis for the long term.[4] Which all sounds pretty good to me, because I love my busy life, and I want to keep adventuring and dancing and creating things for as long as I can.

BRICK HOUSE

I like to hit all of my bases when it comes to building my body. I want to have endurance so that I can go as far and long as I want. I want to be able to keep my balance no mat-

ter what sport I'm playing. I want to keep my muscles flexible and limber. I want the benefits that come with giving my body a chance to explore and expand, to challenge myself, to shock my system, to keep me interested and engaged for the long term.

I also like to vary the time, length, and intensity of my workouts. For example, I might spend one day doing thirty minutes of intense cardio to build endurance, then the next day doing an hour-long low-impact workout (like Pilates or barre) that works my balance and flexibility. Then on the following day I might do forty-five minutes of strength training.

To me, fitness means taking care of your physical body by giving it what it needs at that moment, which changes day by day. Here's a quick lowdown of some of the best ways I know of to help you meet *your* goals.

IF YOU WANT	GO FOR	AND DISCOVER
ENDURANCE	Aerobic exercise—like running, swimming, dancing, spinning, and dance cardio—that uses the large muscles of your body in a rhythmic way over time.[5]	Improved heart and lung strength, which makes your body more resilient to challenges—physical and mental.
STRENGTH	Strength and resistance training using free weights, bands, medicine balls, or body weight (think push-ups)	For women, strength training can help protect against loss of bone mass with age. String muscles also help to keep a body young.
BALANCE	Balance-challenging exercises that make you engage your core muscles to stand up straight, like yoga, barre classes, surfing, and paddle-boarding.	Your sense of balance literally grounds you, helping to protect against falls. It also makes you better at all physical activities.
FLEXIBILITY	Low-impact, muscle-releasing activities—like yoga, Pilates, stretching, warming up before working out, and fascia release (like foam rolling).	Being flexible helps to prevent injuries and improves range of motion. Stretching also speeds recovery after a tough workout.

do
what
feels
good

MIX IT UP

I used to take the same barre class all the time. It was great for working small muscle groups, and the movements helped me feel long and lean. But after a while, I got bored and my body changes plateaued. Because my body stopped changing and I'd grown bored mentally, I knew if I wanted to keep seeing results, it was time to change it up.

Now I try not to adhere to one type of fitness as part of my routine. Every Sunday, I take some time to look at my week and see when I have openings in my schedule. Then I'll try to plug in a different class every day. I might do Pilates on Monday, weight training on Tuesday, dance on Wednesday, spin on Thursday, and barre on Friday. I feel like I've had a comprehensive week when I've worked different muscles than I would have otherwise. I've targeted large muscles and small muscles and burned fat. On the weekend, if I want to go for a run, which I consider more a mental workout for me, that's great. Or I might take a long walk around the city.

It can be tempting to stick with things that we're good at and that feel safe, but with risk comes reward.

If you're just starting out in fitness, you may want to spend some time doing the same kind of workout consistently so that you can really learn and grow and gain confidence. It's okay to embrace a learning curve. You'll know if you get too comfortable and it's time to move on to the next challenge.

A lot of fitness experts out there try to sell you on their "one thing." Whether they're saying yoga is the only way, strength training is best, or their personal brand of dance-cardio is the absolute fastest way to get the body you want, they'll try to convince you that their method is THE most effective way to a better body. This simply isn't true, and we are constantly falling prey to sexy marketing. The reality is, changing things up does a body good.

When you do the same thing over and over again—no matter what it is—your body gets used to it and so does your brain. Your body gets accustomed to working the same muscles and certain movements become ingrained in muscle memory. Instead of exhausting your muscles (and seeing results), you'll hit a plateau. Switching up the muscles that you use every single day creates the best kind of toning for your body. Trying different kinds of sequencing movements also keeps your brain challenged.

There are so many awesome things out there to try. You never know what you might really love! When I started boxing, I discovered that jumping rope is a big part of the sport. Turns out jumping rope is my jam. It took me a few months, but after a while I got better and I even learned how to do some tricks, which really motivated me to keep going. I ended up competing in a jump rope contest, and it was as amazing as it sounds.

As with most things in life, it can be tempting to stick with things that we're good at and that feel safe, but with risk comes reward. I'm not saying you need to stop doing the things you love to keep it feeling fresh. Just change it up incrementally. Bottom line: Change is growth.

GOT THIS GAME IN YOUR HAND

Sometimes I'm motivated to work out because I want to get to a specific class. Sometimes it's really about the afterglow, when I glide through my day feeling energized instead of sluggish. When I'm in a headspace where I'm just not into the idea of working out, I try to remind myself that no matter how hard it is to drag my ass to the gym, I always feel better when I walk out. Here are some of my go-to strategies for staying motivated and not calling in sick (or busy, or tired, or . . .) to my workouts.

remember that you like to feel great. When I'm really not in the mood, I remind myself about all the time I spend with myself outside of class. All the things that I love to do: I can only do them well when I'm in a great state, physically and mentally, and I know that it's my fitness routine that supports my body and mind to be able to do those things.

schedule ahead. Having a plan helps me keep my mind focused. Whatever your schedule looks like, look for opportunities to squeeze in movement. If your workday tends to run long, can you hit the gym before work or at lunch? If you're a freelancer, can you commit to something that adds some more structure to your day? Or can you incorporate fitness into a fun plan with friends? Making a commitment and being held accountable are great motivators.

try something new. I'll always get out of bed for a new kind of fitness opportunity. I believe that varying your routine is an important part of staying motivated, and a big part of my routine is trying new things to keep myself excited and interested.

accept the challenge and embrace the burn. I love a challenge. If your workout feels too easy, something is wrong. Or maybe it's time to step it up to the next level. The fact that exercise is hard and takes discipline and strength is what makes it valuable and translates into skills that transcend the gym. When you feel the burn, that's how you know you're getting somewhere. Pushing past the burn is where you start to see things happen.

know when to go easy. Some days, I might choose a restorative class over something more aggressive because I just need to chill. Other days, my body may express to me that it needs a day off. Like with nutrition, it's so important to tune into your body and listen to its needs. Learning when to go easy makes a routine sustainable. There's a difference between feeling the burn and burning out!

dress the part. Let's be real: Cute clothes are motivating. It's something I experience, and I bet you've experienced it, too. The better I feel in my skin, the more geared up I am for any activity I'm about to engage in. Studies have shown that I'm not the only one who feels this way. *Enclothed cognition* is the term for the way what we wear affects us. Scientists have proven that what we wear has an effect on how we behave when we're engaging in an activity.[6]

It's all about feeling good, so if looking good helps you get there—I say go for it.

#FITNESSGOALS

I've shared what fitness gives me. What do you want it to give you? Understanding what you want to accomplish can help you plan the kinds of fitness you might want to work into your routine. How do you want to feel? Stronger? Faster? More flexible?

I encourage you to set goals that take into consideration where you are now, what is realistic, and what is best for your body. Being inspired by someone else's fitness is a powerful feeling—that's kind of why we watch the Olympics, right? But wanting to *be* someone else is a direct route to feeling bad about yourself. If your goal is to look like Beyoncé—well, only Beyoncé looks like Beyoncé. You've gotta set goals for yourself that are real.

We've all had friends who decide to commit to a new fitness routine but somehow seem to fall off the wagon quickly. Oftentimes that's because they've set wildly unachievable goals. They want to lose ten pounds in a week. They want to have arms like Gwyneth, a butt like Kim, legs like Jourdan. And if they don't see what they want staring back in the mirror, they've failed.

The best fitness goals will be based on *you*. And they don't have to be about waist size. They can be about going further or faster than you did before, gaining strength and flexibility, building more muscle, relieving stress and anxiety. Because I am so into pushing myself, I like to make challenging, measurable goals about my fitness. I set goals to run a lon-

ger distance, to do one more pull-up than last time, or to lift heavier weights. That kind of super-specific, incremental goal setting works for me when I'm planning out my routine for a week or a month, but on any given day my goal might be more about the other qualities of fitness: getting out of a funky mood, listening to music, quieting my mind.

If you're in a stage where you'd like to set some goals for yourself, it can be helpful to use tools to figure out where your body is right now and what it needs given its current state. Maybe that means getting on a scale (or not, if that's not psychologically healthy for you). It could mean going to your doctor for a fitness test or an overall checkup. It could mean taking a food sensitivity test to figure out if your diet is hurting you in ways you might not realize. You might be surprised by the results, and your goals might shift based on what you learn.

Sometimes when I'm working out I'll think to myself, "I bet I can do two classes in a row!" But most of the time, I don't. I stop. I recover. Mind over matter can help you endure some intense situations, but it

> Wanting to *be* someone else is a direct route to feeling bad about yourself.

shouldn't be applied to your daily fitness. The body only needs less than an hour of elevated-heart-rate physical activity each day. If you push yourself too hard, you can go into a state of exhaustion, and your immune system can suffer.

Just like with food, it's important to tune into the wisdom of your body with fitness. In the end, the real goal is to feel at home in your body. If you can figure out your right pace—how many times a week, when to rest, when to stretch, and when to lift, the kind of cardio that really motivates you—I think you'll discover that you have more energy than you did before. That you have gained strength and speed. And that your body is a pretty sweet place to live in, after all.

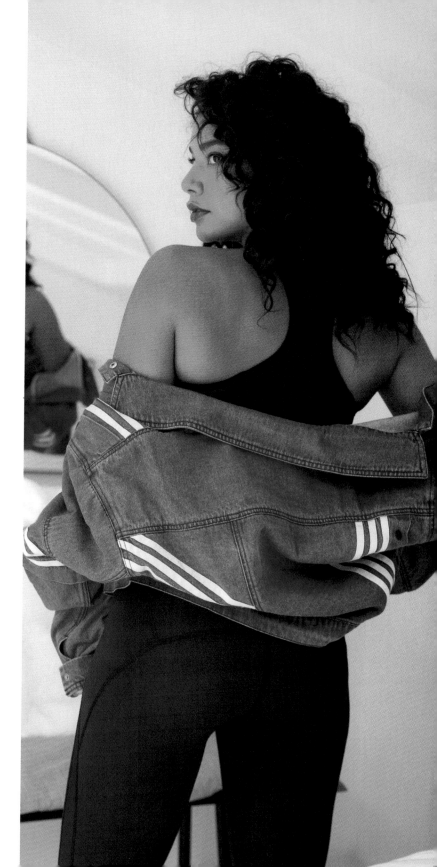

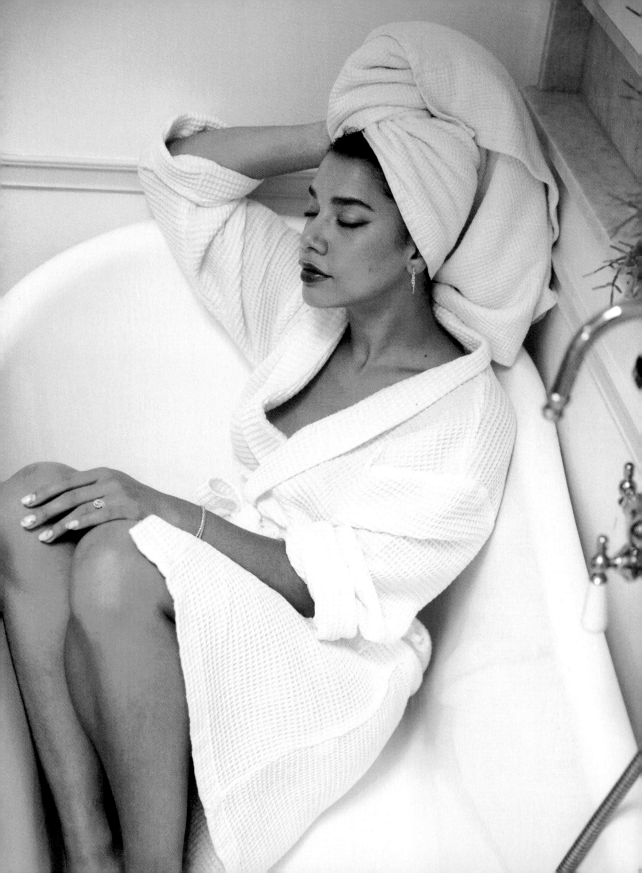

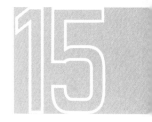

mask ON

HANDMADE BEAUTY AND BATH PRODUCTS

Some people meditate when they want to get in touch with themselves. I know that's something my mom always does. When I need some space to think about what's been going on and have a quiet, reflective moment, I take a bath. I put a mask on my face. I give loving attention to my physical body in order to get closer to my emotions and deeper states of being. I use my quiet time at home, my beauty rituals, to remember that I am always there with myself if I just look close enough.

I bathe around twice a week, and it's my time to chill with myself. Sometimes I light a candle, and I move my phone out of the room because I want to be completely alone and luxuriate in my space with just me and my thoughts as company. Sometimes I have my phone in hand because that's my mood. It's my time, my space, my bath.

I grew up taking baths, and I have a sentimental attachment to the process. When I was a child, my mom would draw me a bath every morning and sing "Wake Up Little

Susie" to me in the bathtub. She would use the handheld shower to suds me up and wash my hair and rinse me clean. It was the best.

As a child, I used to watch a lot of old movies. I always noticed the scenes where people are drawing the heroine a bath. Like when Cleopatra's subjects draw her a milk bath and carry her into the tub like the queen she is. They bathe her and give her a towel afterward, then she would change into some kind of delicate silk outfit. That was my fantasy of being an adult. That and having as many beauty products as I wanted, and using them all, often.

PRODUCT JUNKIE

I have always loved beauty products, ever since I was a kid. I remember going through my mom's bathroom and trying on her perfume, her body lotions. I used my sister's Kiss My Face masks. I would always do those cucumber masks, which made your face burn a little, and then the whole thing would dry and you could peel it off. It was fun, it was new, it was exciting, it was very sensory, and it made me feel good.

Now that I am actually an adult, I get to take all the baths and use all the products I want. Over the years, cleansers, serums, masks, micro rollers, and eye creams have taken a good part of my salary, but it's worth it. Those moments massaging my skin, cleansing, exfoliating, moisturizing, are times when I feel really good. And there is so much on the market to try!!! But however much I love to browse the shelves of Sephora, ultimately I know I probably don't need any more vials, pumps, or jars. At this point I basically have to sneak new products past my husband and into my cabinet. (I know, I know, no man can tell me what to do, but if you saw the way my products have taken over all the cabinets, countertops, and the whole area under the sink . . . you would understand.)

My husband would say I am a beauty junkie, but I say I'm an investigator. I am the ultimate consumer and I love a good brand that meets my needs, but ultimately, I'm always pulling down the curtain and taking a look at what's underneath the hood, so to speak. And as I get older and more serious about taking care of my health, I'm even choosier about what I will put on my skin. That's why I often make my own bath soaks and masks and scrubs out of organic ingredients, and you'll find all of those recipes in a few pages. (Hint: We're not done with avocados yet!)

Just like with my tonics or my food recipes, I love to customize my skin and bath products to my body's needs and my mood, plus I always enjoy making things with my own hands (hence my studying sculpting in college). And knowing that everything I'm about to put on my skin comes from a natural source makes me feel like I'm taking care of myself in the best way. After all, what goes onto your skin gets absorbed *into* your bloodstream, and I care about what's floating around in my blood!

I like to stock up on my favorite natural ingredients—green tea and chamomile tea and honey and coconut yogurt and avocados—so that I always have something on hand to whip up a quick mask or a bath that's a little extra. (And the edible stuff lives in the kitchen, so Brendan can't complain because he ultimately likes his routines, too, even if they are about snacking on my avos.)

With that said, let's get down to the recipes!

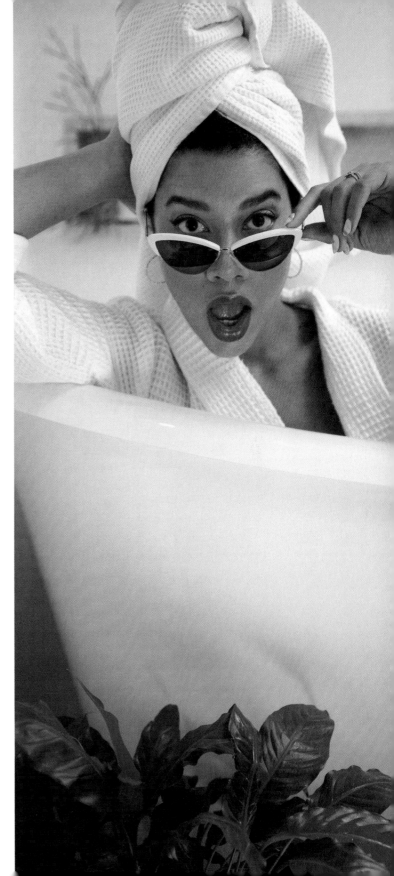

DIY MASKS

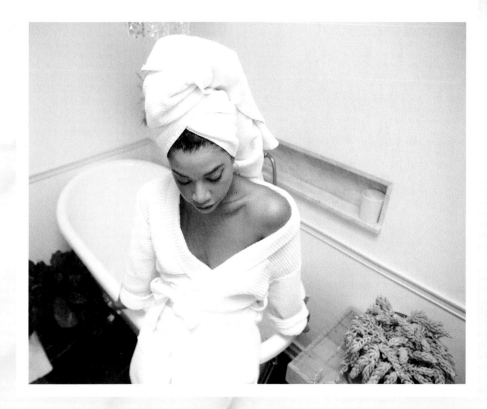

TIGHT AND BRIGHT MASK

Egg white tightens, lemon brightens: This mask is made for skin that's lost its luster. If you're feeling like your skin is looking a little dull, look no further than pearl powder (which you can also drink, like in the Skin Tonic on page 62). When it comes to honey, manuka has the most minerals and nutrients around, and lemons offer vitamin C and citric acid, both of which brighten skin.

INSTRUCTIONS AND USE

1. Blend all the ingredients in a blender, or whip together with a whisk.

2. Apply to the face with a fan brush or your fingers and leave on for 20 minutes.

3. Rinse with lukewarm water and pat dry.

INGREDIENTS

1 egg white whipped

$\frac{1}{2}$ tablespoon raw manuka honey

$\frac{1}{2}$ tablespoon freshly squeezed lemon juice

3 teaspoons pearl powder (see page 62)

HYDRATING MASK 1

INGREDIENTS

1 small organic avocado

1 tablespoon raw coconut yogurt (below)

1 egg yolk

1 tablespoon glycerin

3 drops rose or geranium essential oil

Skin feeling dry? Drink a glass of water and try this avocado-coconut-egg mask, which is all about the moisture. Depending on your scent preferences, you can add rose essential oil, which is so good for hydrating skin, or geranium, which is also wonderful as a skin soother (and priced a little more gently).

INSTRUCTIONS AND USE

1. Blend all of the ingredients to a smooth, velvety consistency in a blender.

2. Apply to the face and let it sit for 20 minutes.

3. Rinse with lukewarm water and pat dry.

RAW COCONUT YOGURT FOR MASKS

You can eat your probiotics, and you can also slather them on your face. And you should! Probiotics make your skin healthier, and healthy skin glows.

INGREDIENTS

1 young Thai coconut

1 to 2 probiotic capsules

INSTRUCTIONS AND USE

1. Blend the coconut water and coconut meat together in the blender.

2. Pour into a mason jar and stir in the powder from the probiotic capsule until the powder is absorbed.

3. Cover tightly with the lid and allow to ferment for 24 to 48 hours.

do
what
feels
good

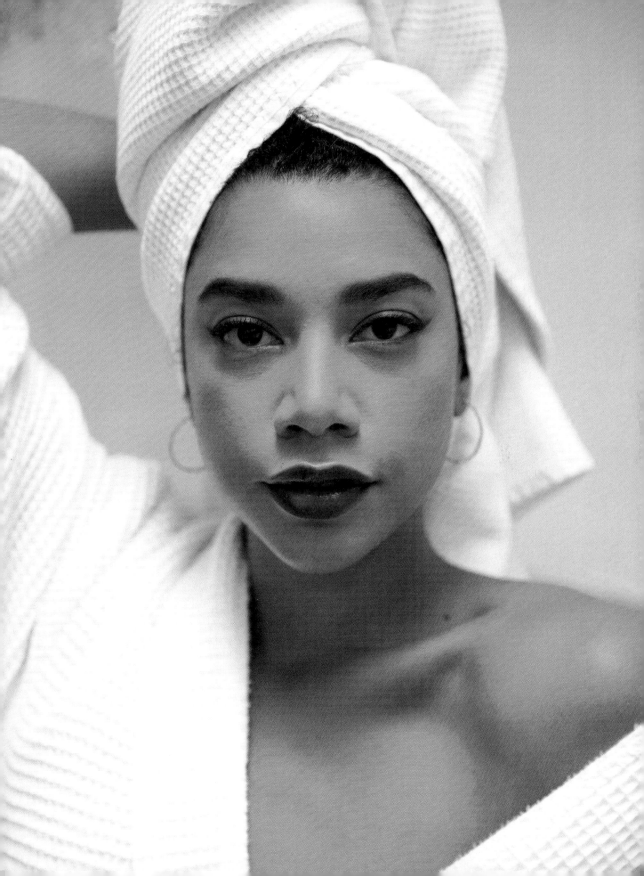

HYDRATING MASK 2

INGREDIENTS

2 tablespoons avocado flesh, at room temperature

1 tablespoon honey

2 tablespoons yogurt (dairy or coconut; see recipe, page 272)

This mask is a slight variation on Hydrating Mask 1—the only difference is that we skip the egg, glycerin, and essential oil and add honey for an ultra-hydrating effect. It feels luxurious on your skin, and it's just the thing if you've spent too much time in the sun or haven't been sticking to your water routine.

INSTRUCTIONS AND USE

1. In a small bowl, mix the avocado with the honey, then mix in the yogurt.

2. Apply to the face and let it sit for 10 minutes.

3. Rinse with lukewarm water and pat dry.

ANTI-INFLAMMATORY MASK

INGREDIENTS

$\frac{1}{2}$ cucumber

2 celery stalks

1 cup yogurt (dairy or coconut; see recipe, page 272)

1 tablespoon fresh mint leaves

2 tablespoons aloe vera gel

1 tablespoon thick raw honey

Sensitive skin sometimes needs a little help to chill out. This cooling mask soothes and smooths with cucumber and celery—two of our beauty foods that also help your skin when you eat them!—mixed with yogurt, mint, aloe gel, and honey.

INSTRUCTIONS AND USE

1. Blend all the ingredients in a blender.

2. Apply to the face and let it sit for 20 minutes.

3. Rinse with lukewarm water and pat dry.

CLAY MASK

If you have oily skin you know it, and you'll appreciate this bentonite clay mask for its clarifying benefits. Witch hazel, honey, and aloe soothe and soften while bentonite does it job of drawing out toxins from the skin.

INGREDIENTS

$1\frac{1}{2}$ tablespoons bentonite clay

1 tablespoon witch hazel

1 tablespoon raw honey

2 teaspoons aloe vera gel

INSTRUCTIONS AND USE

1. In a small bowl, mix all the ingredients with a wooden spoon until well blended.

2. Apply to the face and leave on until the mask starts to tighten.

3. Rinse with lukewarm water and pat dry.

PRO TIP

When you're putting on a mask, don't stop at your chin. Including your neck and your décolletage in the pampering party feels great and nourishes all of the skin that's exposed to the sun on a daily basis.

BEAUTIFYING MASK

INGREDIENTS

2 tablespoons raw coconut yogurt (see page 272)

2 teaspoons raw cacao powder

1 teaspoon kaolin clay

1 teaspoon bentonite clay

1 teaspoon raw honey

1 tablespoon rose water

$\frac{1}{2}$ mashed banana

Raw coconut yogurt and raw cacao blend with two kinds of clay, rose water, and, yes, a banana. Bananas have plenty of vitamin C, which adds a glow to your skin. This mask is great for mature skin, too.

INSTRUCTIONS AND USE

1. In a small bowl, mix all the ingredients together until smooth.

2. Apply to the face and leave on until the mask starts to tighten.

3. Rinse with lukewarm water and pat dry.

GOLDEN MASK

INGREDIENTS

1 tablespoon chickpea flour

2 teaspoons sandalwood flour

1 teaspoon ground, dried turmeric

1 teaspoon neem leaves

2 teaspoons rose water

1 tablespoon raw honey

1 tablespoon melted ghee

1 teaspoon triphala powder

Turmeric is everybody's favorite spice these days. Now you can drink your golden milk and wear it, too, with this golden mask, full of nourishing roots, leaves, and fruits, like healing neem leaf and triphala for skin tone.

INSTRUCTIONS AND USE

1. Add all the ingredients to a blender and blend until smooth.

2. Apply to the face and let it sit for 20 minutes.

3. Rinse with lukewarm water and pat dry.

HAIR AND SCALP CLARIFYING RINSE

Over time, all the products you use leave a layer on your hair and scalp. Changing products helps, and so does this clarifying rinse, made of apple cider vinegar diluted with water. It gives you shinier hair and a cleaner scalp—just keep it out of your eyes!

INGREDIENTS

1 cup water

$\frac{1}{4}$ cup apple cider vinegar

INSTRUCTIONS AND USE

1. Wet your hair thoroughly.

2. Shampoo and rinse your hair as you usually do.

3. Carefully massage in the apple cider vinegar and water mixture and let sit for a few minutes.

4. Rinse, then shampoo and condition your hair as normal.

COFFEE-COCOA BODY SCRUB

I don't drink coffee, but I don't mind smoothing a little caffeine on my arms and legs. Caffeine applied topically helps to reduce inflammation, and this scrub is also an amazing wake-up call, scent-wise. Fair warning: You will probably have to clean your shower after enjoying this one, as it creates a bit of a mess!

INGREDIENTS

1 cup organic coffee grounds

$\frac{1}{2}$ cup organic coconut oil

$\frac{1}{2}$ cup organic macadamia nut oil

30 drops grapefruit essential oil

INSTRUCTIONS AND USE

1. Mix together all the ingredients and store in a mason jar.

2. Apply the scrub to your body in the shower or bath and rinse thoroughly.

3. Moisturize as usual.

ABOUT ESSENTIAL OILS

Essential oils are the carefully extracted essences of fruits, vegetables, herbs, and barks.[1] They've been used basically forever to perfume a stinky world and make everybody look and feel more beautiful. Each oil has its own distinct chemical makeup that lends it properties ranging from antibacterial and antiviral to calming and invigorating.

You'll see these oils in many of my mask and bath recipes. Feel free to play around with them and customize so that you love the scents and can curate a beauty experience made just for you.

I recommend starting with a couple of scents you really love, then adding to your collection as you get to know them. They are generally sold in amber or blue glass to protect them from light. Just make sure to store them in a cool and dark place to keep them fresh and potent. Here are a few of my favorites.

rose oil: The queen of the oils. If you get the real stuff, you'll know because you'll be paying for it. Rose oil is super pricey, has a very deep rose scent, and is magical in body lotions and baths. Also great for skin. Use rose oil when you're in a luxury mood and want to really pamper yourself.

geranium oil: With a floral scent that is very recognizable once you've been introduced, geranium is great for skin and is also known as a hormone balancer for women. Use this oil when you want to chill out.

grapefruit oil: Detox your body and invigorate your mind with this fresh, bright oil. Grapefruit oil is a mood enhancer and can help to reduce water retention—aka bloat.

carrot seed oil: Not the same as carrot oil, which is a base oil, carrot seed oil is an essential oil that fights bacteria and is moisturizing for skin and hair. This one smells super herbaceous, so use sparingly!

fennel oil: Used externally, fennel oil has loads of antioxidants plus antibacterial properties that make it an amazing skin healer.

lemon oil: Made from cold-pressed lemon skins, this oil is energizing and bright. Whatever your skin woes, from acne to aging, lemon oil nurtures, repairs, and hydrates.

cypress oil: Cypress oil has a green, woody scent. It heals wounds and prevents infections.

rosemary oil: This one is an aromatherapy powerhouse, with the ability to lower cortisol and help improve memory. It's also reputed to be amazing for hair growth when rubbed into the scalp.[2]

lavender oil: Lavender is your best friend when you're stressed. And it's so soothing for skin. Add some to your bath, take a few deep breaths, and enjoy the soothing vibe.

valerian oil: Musky valerian is the ultimate chill-out oil. If you want extra relax in your relaxing, try adding a little valerian to your bath.

frankincense oil: A real lifesaver, frankincense oil lowers stress, banishes negative feels, boosts immunity, kills germs—and it's the best, best, best for skin. Acne scars, stretch marks, and dry skin will all benefit from a beauty session that includes some frankincense.

ylang ylang: This oil smells like perfume. It's used as an antidepressant, so if you're feeling stress or anxiety, take a bath with this oil or add it to some unscented lotion for an amazing scented boost. It's also good for skin conditions like eczema.

I GOT BATH WATER YOU CAN SOAK IN

I love a bath, but let's be real: it's not the best way to get clean. Your bath is about soaking and being with yourself. So step one: Shower before you bathe. You want to rinse off your day and all the stuff you may have come in contact with before you climb into the tub. That is not what you want to be soaking in! You want your skin warm and clean to receive and absorb the oils, minerals, salts, and clays that you put in your bath.

Bathing is a ritual that makes you feel good inside and out. When you need to relax, you can have a calming chamomile bath. For extra detox, throw some seaweed in there. If you want to really luxuriate, you can try a coconut milk and honey bath.

When you bathe, try to soak in the warm water for 40 to 60 minutes. You can put on a mask before you get in the tub, and let it absorb and do its magic while you're soaking. But please note that all that soaking can be dehydrating. The warm water can make you sweat, and soaking for too long dries out your skin.

So be careful to hydrate when you bathe: drink water before and after the bath, a big glass each time.

It's also important that you don't rinse off anything you put in your bath. If you have taken the time and care to add oils and clays to your bath, you want your body to soak up all that goodness! Just out of the bath, still damp, is when you'll apply your moisturizer. I usually opt for body oils instead of creams, and sometimes I just use pure coconut oil or shea butter. Whatever you use, make sure you massage it well into your skin to encourage circulation while you sleep.

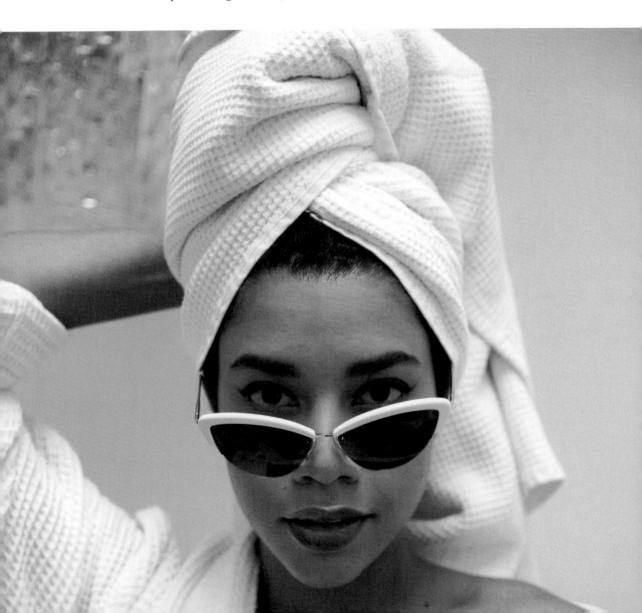

AU REVOIR CELLULITE

A special bath blend to mix and use at your leisure, this is a variation on a recipe from skincare goddess Monica Watters. Beginning your soak with a thorough dry brush (see below) is great for circulation, exfoliates your skin, and can help with the appearance of cellulite. Then come the essential oils: grapefruit to debloat, fennel to minimize fat deposits, and geranium to improve circulation.

INSTRUCTIONS AND USE

1. In a bowl, mix the almond or jojoba oil and carrot seed oil. Add the rest of essential oils and mix. Pour into a glass amber dropper bottle. Drop 10 to 20 drops into your bath.

2. Pour the Epsom salts into the bath.

3. Dry brush your skin from head to toe, then soak.

INGREDIENTS

2 tablespoons almond or jojoba oil

3 teaspoon carrot seed oil

10 drops grapefruit oil

5 drops fennel oil

5 drops lemon oil

5 drops cypress oil

5 drops rosemary oil

5 drops geranium oil

2 cups Epsom salts

DRY BRUSHING

A dry brush is an easy and useful part of a beauty routine, especially before a bath to really get your skin ready for the treats that are coming. You can buy a dry brush online; you're looking for something with natural fibers, not too rough. Hold the brush in your hand and, beginning with your arms, brush your skin gently and firmly, up toward your heart. Then do your legs, moving upward always. It feels great on your back if you can reach or you have someone available to help out. Dry brushing boosts circulation of your blood and of your lymph, and it also exfoliates your skin very nicely.

GREEN TEA DETOX

5 green tea bags

1 cup Epsom salts

Green tea offers powerful antioxidant properties for your insides when taken internally, so why not relax in a green tea bath and give your skin the same anti-aging boost? This is an especially great bath for people who suffer from irritated skin conditions like atopic dermatitis (a type of eczema),[3] as green tea has been found to be soothing for these skin conditions.

INSTRUCTIONS AND USE

1. Steep the green tea bags in 1 cup of hot water for 7 to 10 minutes.

2. Add the tea to your bath along with the Epsom salts.

3. Soak.

EPSOM SALTS

Made of magnesium sulfate, Epsom salts have been used for centuries to relieve aches and pains and soften skin. They are readily available at your drugstore and mix beautifully with any number of herbal or floral additives to help with a multitude of ailments.

do
what
feels
good

EVENING BATH

Chamomile is one of the oldest medicinal herbs around and has been used for ages as a preparation to help people relax and sleep, and to treat the skin. A cup of chamomile tea can soothe your stomach and your nerves;[4] have one and then climb into this sleepy-time bath before bed. I've also added a dose of valerian, which has been shown to decrease beta brainwaves (which are linked to being awake and engaged) while increasing theta brainwaves (which are linked to daydreaming and drowsiness) and delta brainwaves (the brainwaves of sleep and healing).[5,6]

INGREDIENTS

2 chamomile tea bags

1 cup hot water

1 cup Epsom salts

5 drops lavender oil

5 drops valerian oil

INSTRUCTIONS AND USE:

1. Steep the chamomile tea bags in the cup of hot water for 7 to 10 minutes.

2. Add to your bath with the Epsom salts.

3. Soak.

MERMAID BATH

INGREDIENTS

$\frac{1}{2}$ cup dried seaweed (like kelp or dulse), steeped in a cup of boiling water for 30 minutes

$\frac{1}{2}$ cup spirulina

You can let your hair down with this seaweed-enriched soak. Seaweed is hydrating and anti-inflammatory[7] and was used in Japan to wash and condition hair long before commercial shampoo was ever invented. Spirulina is packed with antioxidants and is great for skin taken internally or applied topically, and some research suggests that it can help hair grow when used externally.[8]

INSTRUCTIONS AND USE

1. Strain the seaweed "tea" and pour into your bath.

2. Mix the spirulina in a cup of warm water and add to your bath.

3. Soak.

MILK AND HONEY BATH

INGREDIENTS

1 cup coconut milk powder

2 tablespoons honey

Lift tired skin with a potion reputedly used by Cleopatra, famed legend of beauty and badassery. We've swapped in coconut milk for the mare's milk but kept the honey, which is an antimicrobial that has been used for millennia to heal wounds and fight infection.[9]

INSTRUCTIONS AND USE

1. Add the coconut milk and honey to your bath.

2. Soak like a queen.

do
what
feels
good

SOFTEST SKIN BATH

Dermatologists know that oatmeal has antioxidant and anti-inflammatory properties, and now you do, too.[10] You can find it in commercial preparations, or you can add oat flour to your bath to soothe skin that is dry, itchy, or having an eczema flare-up. Jojoba oil adds extra soothing and softness.

INGREDIENTS

1 tablespoon jojoba oil

$\frac{1}{2}$ cup oat flour

INSTRUCTIONS AND USE

1. Add the oat flour and jojoba oil to your bath.

2. Soak.

PEACE BATH

Spicy frankincense is used as incense for ceremonies, for meditation, and for skin conditions.[11] Ylang ylang is sweet and floral and is known for making you feel relaxed when you inhale it.[12] Blend the two with a few drops of herbaceous lavender and add to your bath for a calming and meditative experience at home.

INGREDIENTS

5 drops frankincense oil

5 drops ylang ylang oil

3 drops lavender oil

1 cup Epsom salts

INSTRUCTIONS AND USE

1. Add all the ingredients to your bath.

2. Soak.

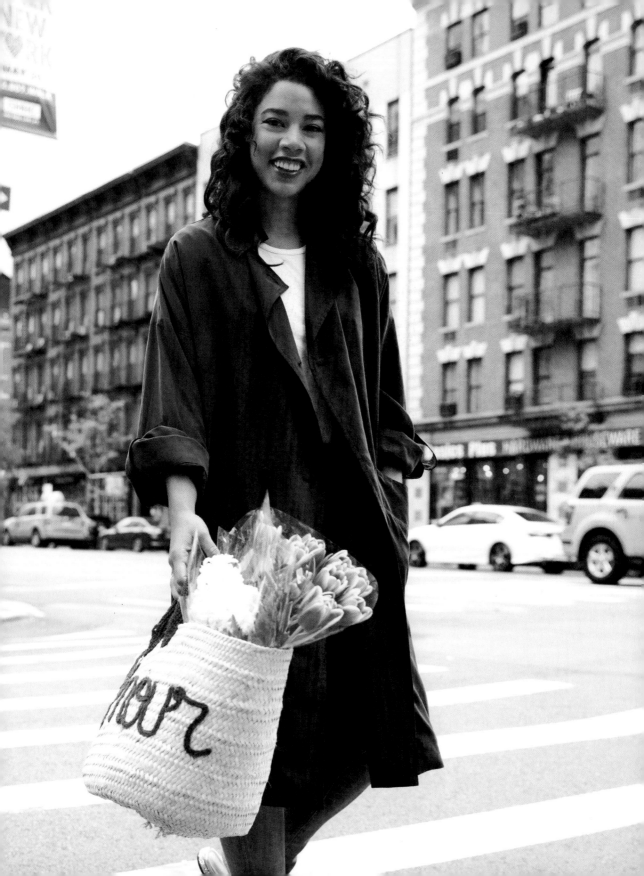

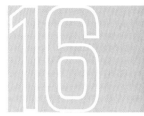

all the ladies IN THE PLACE with style and GRACE

EXPRESS YOURSELF

When I was young, I loved to watch my mother get ready for events. Whether it was a gala or an audition (she was an actress), she always dressed with purpose. I would sit in her room while she got ready, watching the way she selected her clothes and her shoes, the way she put on her face creams and her eye makeup, the way she did her hair just so. When she was done, she was still my mom, but she was someone else, too—someone glamorous, someone powerful, someone invincible. She knew how to make an art out of the process. She would think about what she wanted to express or embody and put herself together accordingly.

In some ways I am just like my mom, and this is one of those ways. What I wear and how I adorn my body completely inform how I feel on my way out the door and ultimately shape the memories I'll make wherever I go.

This idea of your style imprinting your experience of any given moment was never more apparent or relevant to me than when Brendan and I got engaged and began to plan our wedding. I don't think I've ever thought more about clothes than I did when I was wedding planning. It may be a stereotype of any bride-to-be, but I was super aware that every choice I made was going to have an impact on the biggest day of my life—and what I would wear would matter to me in the moment and long after the moment had passed. I mean yes, of course, I wanted to be a beautiful bride, but I also thought a lot about how I wanted to feel, what I wanted to convey, what inspirations I wanted to have around me, what style nods I wanted to give.

My grandmother used to wear an A-line, deep-royal-blue velvet dress with long sleeves and one large white fur pocket on the hip that was very chic and very '40s. I always loved that dress. My dad gave it to me after she died, and it hung in my closet for a while, waiting for the perfect occasion. The dress was so special to me—I knew it was meant for an equally special night.

Brendan and I had planned to have our engagement party in the Seagram's building, which my great-aunt helped design with Mies van der Rohe. The whole thing felt very old-school New York, and very family-centric. So I decided to wear the blue velvet dress as a tribute to my grandmother.

I went to the tailor to customize the dress so that it would fit my curves and height. I turned the skirt into a pencil skirt that hit below my knees with a slit up the back and I shortened the sleeves to a three-quarter length. I wanted to wear it, but I knew that I also needed to feel like myself, to express my style, to have it fit *me*.

When my father saw me he almost cried.

When I think back to that night, the dress is such a vivid part of it all. I felt like my grandmother was smiling on my shoulder the whole evening. All of my memories of that night—the way Brendan looked at me, how excited I felt—are all wrapped in blue velvet.

BEAUTY JOURNEYS

Clothing is transformative. The way we dress affects us emotionally and psychologically. In chapter 15 we touched on the concept of enclothed cognition. A lab coat makes a doctor feel more like a doctor, athletic workout clothes make you feel more athletic, and a full-length gown automatically makes you feel more glamorous. The right gear connects us to who we are and who we want to be. There are some jackets that make you feel like a boss lady telling the world you mean business. There are some dresses that were just made for a night out or that speak to your inner spirit animal. Just like there are some nail colors or textures that were made to go with those dresses. And the mood usually follows along.

Wearing *considered* looks totally influences the vibe of my day or night. By "considered" I mean what I think, what inspires me right now, how I want to feel.

Just putting on something that makes you feel super glamorous can turn a regular day or night into something memorable. Sometimes I get dressed up because I'm feeling spicy, sometimes just because I'm looking to spice things up.

I often DJ events during the week, which means I need to get myself together on a Tuesday or Wednesday night for a huge party. Preparing my look for an event is part of my process. I'll turn on some music and apply a mask while I think about what I'm going to wear. I spend time making sure my hair and makeup feels good because getting my look together puts me in a good mood. If I'm in a good mood, then my energy rubs off on the crowd and that's an important part of being a DJ. The energy that's created with the music is essentially coming from my personal mood. And my style has a huge impact on my mood.

WE NEVER GO OUT OF STYLE

Style is timeless, even though fashion changes over time. When I was a teen I couldn't get enough of tube tops, Lacoste polos, low-cut jeans, and platforms. A few years later I was into the preppy Ab-

ercrombie look. Every season there is another color we are told is the best color, and suddenly every sweater and pair of sneakers and sunglasses comes in that shade. That's fashion.

Style is something else. Style comes from who you are inside as much as from what inspires you or what you think is cool. Developing a personal style is something you can cultivate as you become more aware of yourself and what thrills you and as you encounter more and more things that delight or inspire you. Real style can definitely include the fashions of the day, but it can also include what is vintage, what is creative, what is unusual, because it mostly comes from being at ease with yourself and learning how to express yourself with confidence.

Feeling like we have to be someone else, or to look like someone else, in order to be beautiful, is the opposite of style. Style isn't about being a perfect image of somebody else's perfect image. It's figuring out what fires you up and indulging in it. I used to feel like the way I dressed was all about where I was going and what other people would think of me when they laid eyes on me—would they like me, would I fit in, would I stand out, what would people say? That was related to those periods where I was struggling a lot with self-confidence. That was before I realized that everything I put *in* my body makes me feel a certain way, and that the same is true of what I put *on* my body, in the form of beauty products, and what I dress myself in.

I do not subscribe to the idea of squeezing myself into anything uncomfortable or too small or suffering for a look. If it isn't comfortable, it isn't for me. If it doesn't make me feel good, it isn't for me. What is for me is wearing my heart on my sleeve. I love pieces that remind me of an era I find totally fabulous, or a design that is new and fascinating in a way I haven't really seen around before. As long as it helps me express something I'm feeling or want to feel, I'm down to give it a try.

I swear, magical things start to happen when you wear your confidence as your best accessory. Here are some of my fundamentals of style. I'm sharing them not so you feel like you have to have my style, but to inspire you to find your own personal look that feels empowering and fun. Because being comfortable in your own skin feels really, really good.

- start with a statement: I like to start with one statement piece and build around it. If I've got a pair of pants I've been eyeing, I'll curate a whole outfit around those pants.
- try not to default: It's so easy to fall into jeans and a T-shirt all of the time. Too easy! When I find myself defaulting, I'll reach for a printed blouse that doesn't get enough airtime and use it as the base for a whole different look.

- **make daily luxuries routine:** Style is the end result of doing things that are good for you and make you feel good. Self-care shouldn't be a luxury—it is a requirement.
- **if it feels like you, it's yours:** There's a certain style that's pushed every season—I say wear what you want to wear. There's a certain look that's suddenly everywhere—I say find your own look. Style is not about looking a certain way. It's about feeling a certain way. It's about being free, open, confident, and true to yourself.
- **rock your signature look:** Whether it's a particular shade of lipstick, an eye-catching piece of jewelry, or a great pair of glasses, find one or two signature pieces that scream your name and make them part of your everyday style.

I ROCK TOM FORD

When I was younger, I was a serious nail-biter—it was how I alleviated anxiety and stress. I would gnaw on my cuticles constantly and generally chomp on my fingertips to comfort myself. When I performed as a ballerina, we were always told to match our nail color to our costume—but I never had enough nail to be painted. I used to say I was the president of the NBA—Nail-Biters Anonymous.

I tried all kinds of things to quit my habit, ranging from bad-tasting polish to Tabasco sauce, but nothing seemed to work. The turning point for me came in college. As a sculpture major, I worked with my hands all the time, and between the biting and being covered in clay and paint, they looked disgusting. I was really bothered by looking at them, embarrassed to have other people see them. And I finally thought, "This is crazy. How can I fix this?"

Luckily this was right around the time that gel manicures became popular. I was amazed by this new technology that could give me nails that were too hard to bite through. The local nail salon near my school campus offered decals and stencils—stuff that was affordable and new and fun. For three months, I kept getting manicures and not biting my nails. Making this one simple change was such a shift for me. To someone else, getting your nails done isn't really a big deal. For me, seeing my hands look healthier and more polished (literally) made me feel so much better about myself.

When I moved back to the city, I continued my new manicure routine. I started to get bolder with my nail art, using my nails to express myself the way some girls use makeup. My nails became about telling a story, having a vibe, expressing my style, and generally making me feel good. One year, around Valentine's Day, I walked into a salon named Valley and met a woman named Mei. I asked Mei if she could paint a portrait of my boyfriend, Brendan, on my nail.

Mei asked to see a photo. She looked at it and said, "Sure, I can do that!"

When she was done, not only could *I* tell it was Brendan, anyone could see it. There, on my nail, was a likeness that was perfectly, unmistakably him. I was like, *This is amazing. You are a master painter on the world's tiniest canvas.*

I kept coming back to see Mei, and we started collaborating on nail art concepts. We would do nails that were very theme heavy, like song lyrics turned into emojis (the Jay Z lyrics "I don't pop Molly, I rock Tom Ford" nails were pretty epic). We've

> My nails became about telling a story, having a vibe, expressing my style.

tried all sorts of graphics and all sorts of themes, including Rihanna-inspired champagne-shaped nails for my golden birthday and Hillary Clinton–themed nails (which her campaign re-posted, NBD).

Anyway, I'm sharing my crazy nail journey to illustrate how something that started as an unhealthy habit became one of my favorite forms of self-care. And how you can use even the smallest parts of your personal style to make a statement, one that reflects everything from who you love to who you vote for.

The media tends to hype beauty as a corrective force—cover up this pimple, enhance this feature, hide this flaw, and you will be more attractive to others. It is easy to fall victim to that kind of thinking, to dress in a way that hides the body you have, to groom yourself in a way that conceals the features that make you unique. Now I know that makeup and clothes and accessories and all other types of adornment are best worn to express yourself, not hide yourself. Showing off who you really are begins with understanding who you are.

There's nobody out there that can do me more authentically than I can do me.

There's nobody out there who can do you more authentically than you can do you.

GIRL WITH A DRAGON TATTOO

If you ask a black girl about her hair, you're not going to get a simple answer. Because it is complicated—really complicated.

It's taken me a long time to understand my hair, and to understand my relationship with my hair. Over the years, my hair has gone through many phases. I relaxed my hair when I was a teenager. I would blow it out for any occasion. It wasn't until I was in college that I started wearing my hair natural, but I still didn't embrace a totally natural style. I would wash it and air-dry it and then straighten the roots and put it up. I didn't embrace the curl.

Then, when I was twenty years old, my best friend got a tattoo. She asked if I would come with her and, of course, I did, not realizing that this simple trip to Woodstock would lead to a revolutionary decision. Growing up, I had always been the girl who never wanted any tattoos. But while my friend consulted with a tattoo artist, I started idly flipping through the book of art. Mermaids, anchors, cartoons, snakes, skulls, dragons, basically anything you could think of was on display in these books. The drawings were beautiful. And suddenly, there I was, considering a tattoo.

"Maybe I could get one on the bottom of my foot?" I said to the artist who was working on my friend. It would be my little secret.

"What would be crazy is if you would shave your head and get a tattoo on your skull!" said the artist.

"What!!?" I said.

Turned out her husband had started a tat on his head but couldn't finish it because it hurt too much. She said, "Why don't you just keep looking at some inspiration and if you're inspired by something and want to go through with this I'll do it for free?"

I made the appointment for the following week, knowing that if I didn't show up, no harm, no foul.

A week went by and I woke up to eight of my girlfriends hovering over me. My friend (the same one who had gotten the tattoo the week before) led the charge and insisted that she was shaving my head. Suddenly we were in my bathroom having a total rebel moment. Just like that, a third of my hair was gone.

It was on.

I had already picked out the tattoo: a dragon head with a body made of a vine

(a flower vine), in the shape of a seahorse, which fit the curvature of my head. It took them seven and a half hours to tattoo my head, and it was the most painful thing I've ever done. I took one thirty-minute break between the outline and filling it in. I was whimpering and crying the whole time, but it was one of those things that I just had to see through. I had all my girlfriends with me for moral support, and they really helped.

When the artist was finished, one side of my head still looked the way it always had, and the other side was pale, bald, and covered in this huge tattoo. When I caught my reflection in the mirror, it felt like everything would be different forever.

The first time my mother saw my new look, she was silent for a moment, taking it all in. And then she finally spoke: "Well, at least you chose the only place on your body that doesn't sag." We both laughed, and I was relieved that she wasn't mad. But as we started to talk about it, a deeper conversation evolved that taught me a few things.

My mother told me that if she had done something like this when she was my age, her mother would have killed her. Growing up black in Chicago in the '50s meant that your dresses needed the proper stitch to show you were socially acceptable, that you weren't poor, so my mother learned how to sew and hand-made her clothes. She was told her hair needed to look more like white people's hair. If you were black and wanted to move up in the world, it was important that you didn't look too black. It was important to conform to a white standard of beauty.

And there I was, half a century later—feeling a mix of rebelliousness, empowerment, and pressure. Once I was out of school and started my professional life, that rebellious streak subsided and I didn't embrace my natural hair. For whatever reason I just felt it wasn't elegant, it wasn't polished. That it wasn't going to make me feel professional or that I may not be taken seriously. For years we've been told that if you are a professional woman you need to look a certain way, basically basic: always the same simple and boring look. I feel like we are constantly told that the expressive individual is not going to excel in the workplace. So I conformed, for a while (at least when it came to my hair).

It's only very recently that people have started to embrace women and women of color and individual style in the workplace. It's part of the journey of this country, as we look for identity. It's wonderful to see that conversations are changing and moving toward embracing individuality rather than uniformity. But it's still a work in progress. We are, thankfully, starting to get to another layer of the conversation: that we need to stop pretending we are all the same. It is our individuality that makes America beautiful. It's work that is crucial because we all deserve to love what we see in the mirror, and not to live in a society that tells us that there is only one kind of beautiful, only one look that says smart or educated or professional or acceptable.

The long road to accepting my natural hair is part of a much longer journey to self-acceptance and confidence. After all, style is a form of self-expression. And before you can decide what you want to wear, or how to do your hair, you have to know who you are.

BRAIDED BEAUTY

Accepting my hair was one thing. Embracing it is another. As I was writing this book, it dawned on me that I've been playing myself for thirty years. I now realize that the looks I once saw as risk-taking or adventurous have actually been pretty safe. I haven't veered far from the standards of beauty created by white America.

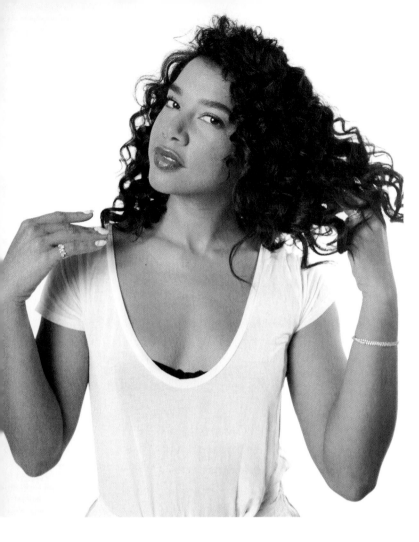

and enjoy the process of playing with my hair, of doing my hair for a meeting or a night out, but not feeling trapped by one idea of how I should look. For a black woman, the way you choose to wear your hair is a big deal. The way I choose to wear my hair on any given occasion is an expression of how I feel, how I see myself, how I want you to see me. There's a lot of power in that when it comes from a place of ease and comfort, but it can take time to let go of other people's shitty ideas, the ones that you've been absorbing for years. The belief that you've got to look *other than you are* in order to do well in this world. Now I want to start absorbing some better ideas, like these: Individuality makes us powerful. Heritage and culture are essential parts of ourselves that we shouldn't erase to make other people feel more comfortable.

It isn't always easy to see where we've been railroaded, and it amazes me how something like hair is really attached to so much trauma that I just accepted as normal for so long. Which means that when

Now I'm trying to find another part of myself—a part that has always been there, a part that I am excited to celebrate.

After all the blowouts, relaxers, haircuts, and, yes, the tattoo, I am finally saying fuck it. I'm giving my natural hair a spin. And I'm loving it.

I'll be honest, it's a lot of work—my hair can have multiple personalities—but it's also fun to embrace the versatility. I'm trying to get to a place where I can be creative we unpack our feelings around certain styles, we can gain a lot of self-awareness and grow as people.

Recently, when prepping and practicing my pre-vacation self-care routine before taking an anniversary trip to a very humid island, I thought about how I didn't want to deal with taking care of my hair or bringing a ton of products that would explode in my bag. Obviously, we all use Instagram as a tool for inspiration, and as a good algorithm does, it was serving me up all sorts of braided brown beauties on my explore page.

"I want to do that!" I thought.

But something stopped me from making an appointment to get my hair braided. I wanted to have a cool hairstyle, and yet I was scared to go through with it. All of these negative feelings came up for me. Things that I heard in my youth, like you're not black enough to do that or braids aren't becoming of a respectable girl. Were these the voices of friends, strangers, authorities, media? Or just purely what I observed? All of these feelings came up for me. I couldn't believe that I was being such a baby about getting my hair braided. Even saying it was for a vacation felt like I was looking for excuses or reasons why it was okay to just get some braids.

I imagined what would happen if I put a photo of myself in braids on Instagram. I immediately thought of the negative comments that might appear. I pride myself on my style and my self-expression, and here I was, feeling so vulnerable and anxious. In my mind I was transported back to the days when I was a teenager and felt like I had to constantly prove myself to everyone.

Back then, I was a bit of a troublemaker. I always wanted to do things my way, and as you can imagine, my teachers and my parents weren't into my behavior. When they said, "No you can't," I said, "Yes I can." There's still a part of me that wants to prove myself, and I've gotten good at using it as fuel for getting ahead. It's my fire and my motivation. When I remember that there are people who think I shouldn't, it makes me want to do it all the more.

So I did the damn thing.

I went with medium-thickness box braids and picked out a few accessories— some charms and some gold string that was wrapped around a few braids. I loved how I looked. It was different from anything I had ever felt before. Not only did I feel like the braids suited me, but they also made me feel empowered. Powerful.

The world is obsessed with women's appearances: with the shape of our bodies, with our skin color, with how pretty we can make ourselves in a way that attracts and doesn't offend. What I have learned from my beauty inspirations and from my own beauty trials is that it isn't your job NOT to offend people. It's your job to celebrate you.

NATURAL MYSTIC

Have you ever met somebody who just truly, fully lives within themselves? These are the people who can wear the weirdest outfits and look radiant. They can always pull "it" off, because what they're showing you is themselves.

Anytime I meet someone who has that kind of natural style and self-confidence, I feel inspired. There's something so beautiful about a woman who has no desire to conform, someone who is comfortable expressing herself regardless of how she is judged or perceived. I think we can all learn something from that. I know I can.

How we look affects how we feel. It's all connected: Feeling good is an inside-out job, and it's also an outside-in kind of thing. What I eat and how I move affect mood, and my mood is reflected in my style, the beauty products I use, how often I give myself the luxury of a nice long contemplative soak in the tub. That kind of self-care makes me feel lifted so that I'm inspired to care about the way I present myself to the world. The energy from the looks I create powers me through my days and nights. The good feelings from those experiences give me energy to keep taking care of my health. And, I hope, the energy I put out there affects the people around me in positive ways, too. It's all one big relational circle, and it all matters.

At the end of the day, everything we've talked about here—the self-care, the skincare, the fashion, the hair, the hydration, the sweaty workouts, the avocado-on-everything—is part of a larger cultural conversation about wellness. And yes, it's easy to dismiss it all as a lifestyle trend, but I see this conversation as something meaningful. There is power in women sharing knowledge with one another. There is power in being vulnerable. There is power in talking honestly and openly about our physical and mental health, and in sharing the practices that make us feel good. I hope that this book serves to continue that conversation, and to support and lift you on your own journey to feeling your best.

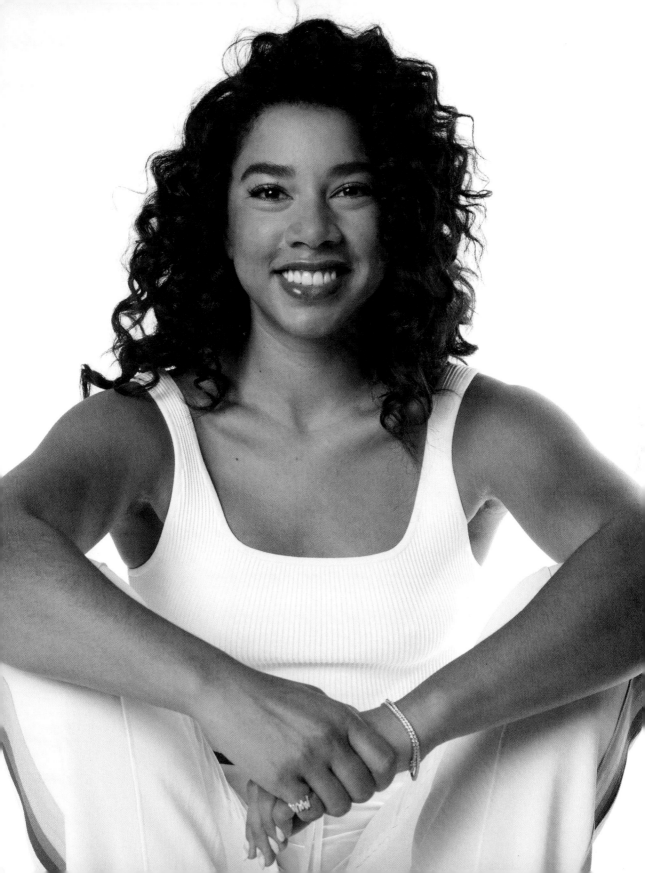

Acknowledgments

I have to start by saying that, Mom, you have been my biggest cheerleader and supporter since day one. I don't know where I would be without your guidance and knowledge. Your health and self-discovery journey has been so inspiring to me! Even when I was a little girl and would sneak into the kitchen during your meditation, you somehow always knew I was there staring at you! I thought you had magic powers, and I now realize that you are simply magic. I want to thank my whole family for having my back and always holding me accountable for my actions, while also teaching me that execution is more important than saying you will do something. To my sisters, thank you for allowing me to lead by example and for always coming to me with your feelings, good or bad. To my rock and favorite human, my husband, Brendan, thank you for always striving to keep me thinking outside the box and consistently reminding me that I can do anything.

To my manager, Gabe Walker, the most opinionated and hardworking man on the planet, I feel so lucky to have you by my side. You make me want to work harder and better than even I think is humanly possible. Tamar, thank you for handling the role of twelve people at all times. You are a wonder woman, and I am so grateful to have you on my team. To my amazing team at WME, Ben Simone and Strand Conover, you guys are always championing me and constantly helping me grow. Margaret Riley King, thank you for understanding my vision and helping me shop this book so that we found the best partner to really let me do it my way! To my legal team at Reed Smith, Ed Shapiro and Sahra Dalfen, thanks for making sure I am always protected.

Of course, none of this would be possible without my amazing publisher, Harper-Wave, who believed in me, helped me shape my story, and brought this baby to life! Specifically, my incredible editor, Julie Will, whose eyes have read this book as much as my own. Julie, you have shown me that you can read page after page, have a little one at home, and still get it all done (of course, with the help of assistant editor Haley Swanson!). Inspiring!

Joanne O'Neill and Bonni Leon-Berman, thank you for making this book look and feel like me! To my publicity gurus, Chelsea Thomas and Alexandra Croton, thank you for believing in my vision and where I'm looking to take my career while also always having my back. To the amazing PR and marketing team at HarperWave, Yelena Nesbit and Penny Makras, thank you for helping me get the word out on *Do What Feels Good*. It's my baby and I appreciate your direction, experience, and guidance on the best way to get this book into everyone's hands and hearts! Also, a big thank you to my production editor, Nate Knaebel.

As you know, I am a very visual person, and the photos in the book needed to reflect me and my passion for storytelling, so I want to thank everyone who contributed to that process. Julia Choi and Evi Abler, thank you so much for making my recipes come to life! Kelsey Cherry and Nolan Knight, thank you for getting my best angles and making this process seamless!

Last, but certainly not least, to my glam team, Takisha and Bob, thank you for always making me feel good in the skin I'm in.

Notes

CHAPTER 2: LISTEN TO YOUR BODY: YOUR SKIN TELLS A STORY

1. https://www.self.com/story/beautiful-skin-superfood-blueb, accessed June 10, 2018
2. https://www.livestrong.com/article/408875-the-best-vegetables-for-good-skin/, accessed June 10, 2018
3. http://www.health.com/health/article/0,20411530,00.html, accessed June 10, 2018

CHAPTER 3: LOVE YOU, MEAN IT: SELF-CARE STARTS WITH YOUR GUT

1. https://www.theatlantic.com/health/archive/2015/06/gut-bacteria-on-the-brain/395918/, accessed May 3, 2018
2. https://www.ncbi.nlm.nih.gov/pmc/articles/PMC4425030/, accessed
3. https://www.webmd.com/skin-problems-and-treatments/guide/what-is-candidiasis-yeast-infection#1, accessed May 21, 2018
4. https://www.healthline.com/nutrition/candida-symptoms-treatment, accessed May 21, 2018
5. https://www.liverfoundation.org/for-patients/about-the-liver/health-wellness/, accessed

CHAPTER 4: THE POTION PROJECT: TONICS FOR HIGHER VIBES

1. https://www.livestrong.com/article/269199-caffeine-effects-on-the-adrenal-function/, accessed June 10, 2018
2. https://draxe.com/mct-oil/, accessed May 22, 2018
3. https://www.vogue.com/article/pearl-powder-skin-food-supplements-amanda-chantal-bacon, accessed February 16, 2018
4. https://www.ncbi.nlm.nih.gov/pmc/articles/PMC5198446/, accessed February 15, 2018
5. https://www.livestrong.com/article/359649-horsetail-extract-its-benefits-side-effects/, accessed May 4, 2018

6. https://www.mountainroseherbs.com/products/shatavari-root-powder/profile, accessed May 4, 2018

7. http://www.dragonherbs.com/prodinfo.asp?number=448, accessed February 16, 2018

8. https://www.webmd.com/vitamins-supplements/ingredientmono-785 -COLOSTRUM.aspx?activeIngredientId=785, accessed February 16, 2018

9. http://thechalkboardmag.com/superfood-spotlight-he-shou-wu, accessed May 3, 2018

CHAPTER 5: EVERYTHING'S BETTER WITH ALMOND BUTTER: EAT WHAT FEELS GOOD

1. https://www.ewg.org/foodnews/, accessed April 29, 2018

2. https://www.nongmoproject.org/gmo-facts/, accessed April 29, 2018

3. http://www.health.com/health/article/0,20480417,00.html, accessed April 29, 2018

4. https://draxe.com/free-range-chicken/, accessed April 29, 2018

5. https://www.womenshealthmag.com/food/a19937556/farm-raised-salmon -healthy/, accessed April 29, 2018

6. https://draxe.com/benefits-of-dark-chocolate/, accessed May 10, 2018

7. https://www.healthline.com/nutrition/9-proven-benefits-of-almonds#section1, accessed May 11, 2018

8. https://www.organicfacts.net/health-benefits/seed-and-nut/health-benefits-of -cashews.html, accessed May 11, 2018

9. https://www.healthline.com/nutrition/13-ways-sugary-soda-is-bad-for -you#section2, accessed May 10, 2018

10. https://draxe.com/nutritional-yeast/, accessed May 10, 2018

11. https://health.usnews.com/wellness/food/articles/2016–10–28/5-reasons-to -start-eating-full-fat-dairy-according-to-science, accessed April 29, 2018

CHAPTER 7: BROTH FOR DAYS: SOUPS AND OTHER LIQUID MAGIC

1. https://www.shape.com/healthy-eating/cooking-ideas/8-reasons-try-bone-broth, accessed May 9, 2018

2. https://www.ars.usda.gov/plains-area/gfnd/gfhnrc/docs/news-2013/dark-green -leafy-vegetables/, accessed May 9, 2018

CHAPTER 12: HEALTHY HEDONISM: DESSERTS AND SOMETHING EXTRA

1. https://www.bonappetit.com/story/what-is-cacao, accessed May 17, 2018

2. https://www.epicurious.com/ingredients/different-types-of-cocoa-powder -recipes-article, accessed May 17, 2018

CHAPTER 14: #FITFAM: GET UP AND MOVE (BUT REST DAYS, TOO)

1. https://www.health.harvard.edu/blog/regular-exercise-changes-brain
    -improve-memory-thinking-skills-201404097110, accessed May 8, 2018
2. https://www.ncbi.nlm.nih.gov/pmc/articles/PMC3448908/, accessed
3. https://www.ncbi.nlm.nih.gov/pubmed/26248288, accessed
4. http://time.com/4776345/exercise-aging-telomeres/, accessed
5. https://www.cdc.gov/physicalactivity/basics/glossary/index.htm, accessed
6. https://www.sciencedirect.com/science/article/pii/S0022103112000200,
    accessed February 18, 2018

CHAPTER 15: MASK ON: HANDMADE BEAUTY AND BATH PRODUCTS

1. https://draxe.com/essential-oil-uses-benefits/, accessed June 15, 2018
2. https://draxe.com/rosemary-oil-uses-benefits/, accessed June 15, 2018
3. https://www.ncbi.nlm.nih.gov/pmc/articles/PMC3408302/, accessed February
    15, 2018
4. https://www.ncbi.nlm.nih.gov/pmc/articles/PMC3408302/, accessed February
    15, 2018
5. Schulz H., Jobert M., Hiibner W.D. The quantitative EEG as a screening
    instrument to identify sedative effects of single doses of plant extracts in
    comparison with diazepam. Phytomedicine. 1998;5:449–458. doi: 10.1016/
    S0944–7113(98)80041-X.
6. https://www.scientificamerican.com/article/what-is-the-function
    -of-t-1997–12–22/, accessed February 15, 2018
7. https://www.womenshealthmag.com/beauty/5-nourishing-seaweed-products,
    accessed February 15, 2018
8. http://www.stylecraze.com/articles/best-benefits-of-spirulina-for-skin-hair-and
    -health/#gref, accessed February 16, 2018
9. https://www.ncbi.nlm.nih.gov/pmc/articles/PMC3609166/, accessed February
    15, 2018
10. https://www.ncbi.nlm.nih.gov/pubmed/22421643, accessed February 15,
    2018
11. https://www.mountainroseherbs.com/products/frankincense-essential-oil
    /profile, accessed February 15, 2018
12. https://www.mountainroseherbs.com/products/ylang-ylang-essential-oil/profile,
    accessed February 15, 2018

Index

C

Golden Mask, 276
Golden Toddy, 212
grapefruit oil, 278, 281
grass-fed cattle, 85
Greek yogurt:
    Digestion Smoothie, 46
    Greek Yogurt Pancakes, 106
    Pro Smoothie, 43
    Spice-Rubbed Salmon with Cucumber-Yogurt Sauce, 161
    Sumac Lamb and Yogurt Bowl, 161
Green Bowl with Chicken, Citrus, and Herbs, 151
Green Detox Soup, 134
Green Goddess Dressing, 90, 152, 168, 176, 186
green tea, 32
    Detox Support Smoothie, 44
Green Tea Detox, 280, 282
Supercharged Matcha Latte, 57
Very Green Ginseng Soup, A, 129
grocery lists, 80
gut health, 178
    body signals and, 37–38
    clear skin and, 7, 25–27
    Detox Support Smoothie, 44
    Digestion Smoothie, 46
    glow foods and, 32
    good gut food and, 41–42
    juicing and, 42
    microbiomes and, 38–39, 40
    pre- and probiotic foods for, 40–42
    Pro Smoothie, 43
    yeast infections and, 39–40
    see also digestive system

H

habits, awareness of, 246–47
Hair and Scalp Clarifying Rinse, 277
hash:
    Bacon, Onion, and Potato Hash, 89, 118
    Baked Eggs in Hash, 119
    Sweet Potato Hash, 117
HBFIT, health journey of, 1–7, 34, 50–51, 242–43
healthy cooking, 73–75
    see also individual recipes
healthy eating, 3, 31–33, 76–80
    see also food shopping
healthy fats, 32, 169
Herbs and 'Shrooms Frittata, 114
herbs and spices, 89–90
    basil, 89, 115, 130, 144
    cayenne, 89, 179
    cinnamon, 46, 61, 89
    dill, 90, 168
    mint, 89–90, 130
    nutmeg, 89, 107, 226–27
    rosemary, 89, 118, 179, 188
    za'atar, 152, 172
    see also ginger
hormonal balance, 7, 28, 32, 34, 53, 278
Hot Honey, 212
hydration:
    beauty masks for, 272–74
    healthy routines for, 242–46
    when bathing, 280, 284

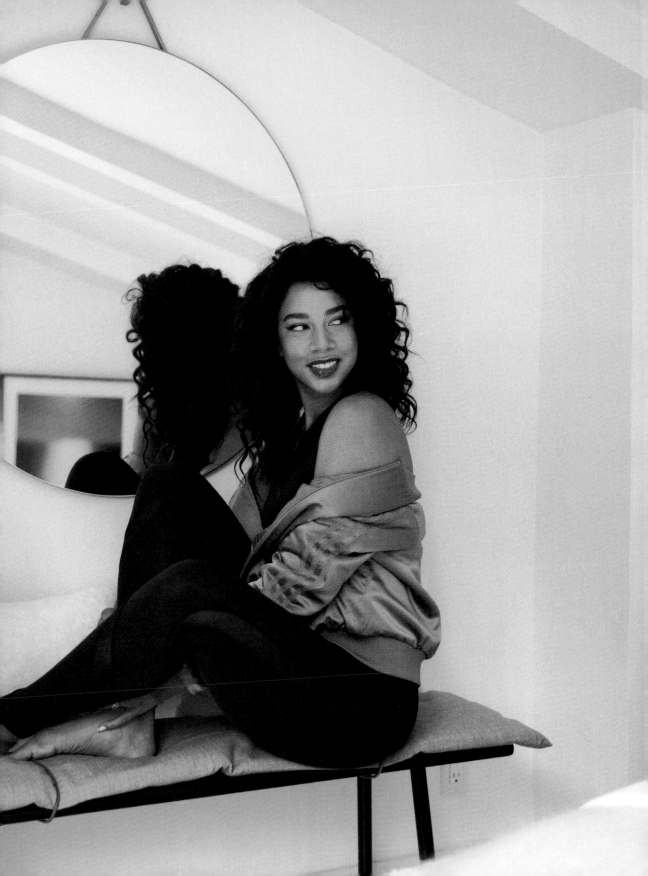

About the Author

Hannah Bronfman is a DJ, on-camera personality, entrepreneur, and wellness enthusiast. She received her MFA from Bard College and is the founder of HBFIT, a unique destination for exploring all things health, beauty, and fitness. She lives with her husband in New York City.

HarperCollins books may be purchased for educational, business, or sales promotional use. For information, please email the Special Markets Department at SPsales@harpercollins.com.

FIRST EDITION

Designed by Bonni Leon-Berman

All food photography and photographs of the author on pages 47, 48, 96, 105, 124, 150, 162, 181, 194, 204, 211, and 223 copyright © Evi Abeler; all other photographs of the author copyright © Kelsey Cherry.

Endpaper illustration by Ali McDonald

Library of Congress Cataloging-in-Publication Data has been applied for.
ISBN 978-0-06-279095-8

19 20 21 22 23 LSC 10 9 8 7 6 5 4 3 2 1

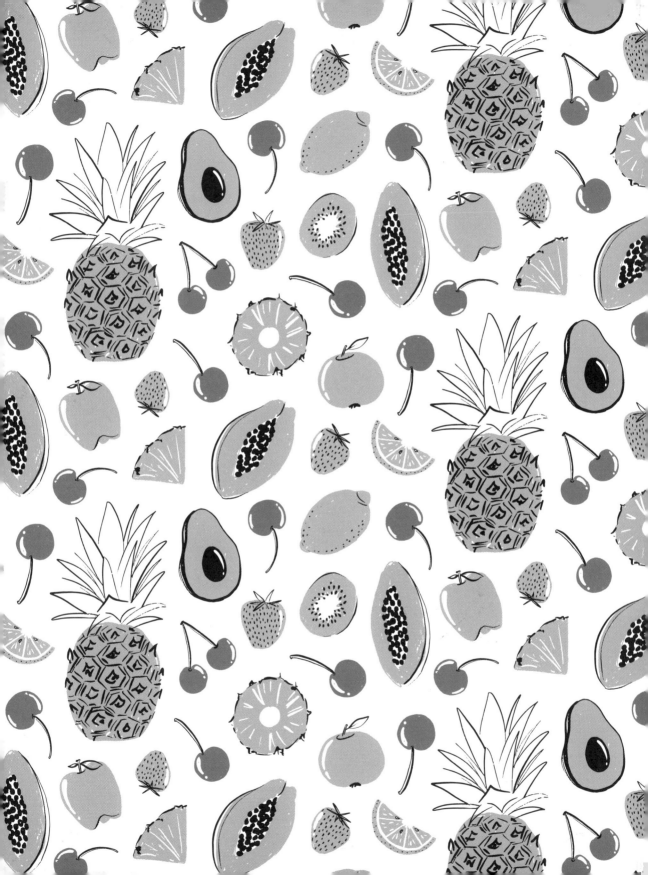